Building Muscle for Beginners

The Foolproof Method for Creating the Perfect Male Body (2022 Guide for Newbies)

Doug Weber

Table of Content

INTRODUCTION

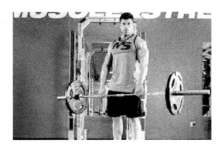

"No man has the right to be an amateur in physical training." It is a pity for a man to grow old without seeing the beauty and strength of his body." - Socrates.

Who would have guessed that one of history's greatest thinkers would be as passionate about physical training as he was about philosophy and contemplation? You can't deny that he has a compelling case here. Our very existence as humans is a miracle in and of itself. Consider how many possible determinants had to be met for you to arrive here - to be who you are right now. It's almost incomprehensible in terms of mathematics. It would be a terrible waste of your life if you didn't push yourself to see how far you can go; how much you can endure; and how much you can accomplish.

It's a good thing if you want to have a chiseled and muscular frame. You are not shallow or pretentious in your desire to look good and have a better build. When someone tells you that obsessing over building your body is shallow, remind them that you have Socrates on your side, and that man was far from shallow. You comprehend the journey you wish to undertake. It's about more than just getting bigger biceps or a more sculpted chest. It all comes down to what these physical manifestations represent. It's all about the effort and dedication you put into achieving your goals. By picking up this book, you demonstrate to yourself and the rest of the world that you are a curious soul eager to learn. You're demonstrating that you're not afraid to go after what you want. That is always the first step toward becoming a better version of yourself than you were yesterday.

Of course, motivation to do good and make a difference is essential. Something of yourself is insufficient. You also need the know-how and the proper game plan to get from where you are to where you want to go.

You've arrived at your destination. That is exactly what this book will assist you with. When you look at the world's elite athletes and see their prime bodies that look like the gods themselves sculpted them, it's easy to become discouraged and believe that you'll never be able to compete. However, you must remember that all of these elite athletes began somewhere. Many of them may have started in worse shape than you are right now. The only thing separating you from them is the amount of work they've already done. Fortunately, there is still time for you to do everything necessary to achieve your desired body. This book will help to illuminate the art of bodybuilding and the science behind it. It is critical that you gain a basic academic understanding of how your body works and what you need to do to care for it. This book will also go over the roles of exercise and nutrition and how you can use these tools to shape your ideal body.

physical shape Most importantly, this book will provide you with all of the fundamental information you need to chart your course in the future. At the end of the day, everyone's bodies are all different shapes and sizes. This is why you must be able to create a plan for yourself that is tailored to your specific needs and goals. Don't be concerned. It's not as difficult as it appears. This book will guide you through the entire process in a very structured and purposeful manner, avoiding any misunderstandings about what to do to achieve your goals. However, in addition to discussing what this book is, it is also important to emphasize what this book is not.

First and foremost, this book will not do your work for you. Reading this book does not automatically guarantee that you will get the body you desire. The most important step here is to apply your knowledge to your daily life to the best of your ability. This book will not provide you with a one-size-fits-all solution to all of your problems. Recognize that every person is unique. A training plan designed for an elite athlete may not always be effective for a novice or beginner. This book, on the other hand, can provide you with enough information and perspective to understand the potential and limitations of your own body. It makes no difference if you're overweight, differently abled, or whatever. It makes no difference if you are gluten intolerant or diabetic. All of the principles presented in this book can still assist you in your fitness journey. The Advantages of Lean and Healthy Muscle

Building

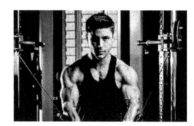

To give you even more motivation to work hard on your muscle-building goals, you should know that the benefits of your efforts go beyond mere aesthetics. It's not just about how your body will appear on the outside. Sure, knowing you look good can make you feel great. However, many of the advantages can also be found on the inside. Sure, many diehard bodybuilders will tell you that being able to achieve their goals brings them a lot of joy and fulfillment.

The fulfillment you receive is a benefit in and of itself, but it is also so much more. Sure, weight training is primarily concerned with muscle building, but there are other physical benefits to strength training as well. This is a common misconception about people who want to build muscle. Here are just a few of the numerous applications of construction.

Muscle can help you have a higher quality of life: Muscles Aid in Blood Sugar Control. Muscles do not, by themselves, regulate the body's blood sugar levels. Rather, the resistance training required for bodybuilding aids in the regulation of the body's blood sugar levels. Many doctors advise anyone with Type 2 Diabetes to engage in resistance or anaerobic training. This is because strength training improves your body's ability to process glucose and deliver it to the muscle, lowering your blood sugar levels at any given time.

Muscles Aid in Body Fat Control

Muscles are known to help control your body fat levels by increasing your metabolism. Metabolism is the process by which your body converts stored fat into energy for movement and bodily functions. As a result, the more muscles you have, the more energy your body requires to function. The more energy you expend, the more fat you burn. Bulking up is more than just getting sculpted. It's also about losing that stubborn fat, which is a leading cause of disease in many people.

Muscles Increase Functional Strength

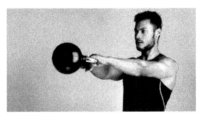

Resistance training makes you bigger and stronger, but it also allows you to lift heavier weights at the gym. All of this increased strength and functionality can be applied to your daily life as well. When you are a stronger person, life becomes easier in general. Lifting heavy boxes will not be a problem when you move. You won't have to worry about trying to pull yourself up onto something. The exercises you do at the gym translate to better movement efficiency in everyday life. However, this may also imply that your friends will contact you first if they require assistance lifting something heavy.

Muscles lower the risk of cancer and heart disease. Muscles, as previously stated, help control the amount of fat in your body. Not all fats, however, are created equal.

Visceral fat is a type of fat that can be extremely harmful to your health. Visceral fat is fat that accumulates on top of your major organs. All of this extra fat can put undue strain on your organs, potentially causing them to malfunction.

This means that your major organs, such as your heart, liver, or kidneys, may be compromised, resulting in serious illness. Furthermore, visceral fat is notorious for promoting the development of cancerous tissues. By engaging in regular strength training, you reduce your chances of developing harmful visceral fat.

Muscles help to strengthen the bones, ligaments, and joints. Having bigger and stronger muscles will help you be a more durable person in general. This is especially useful if you are an athlete who enjoys staying active. For example, if you are a long-distance runner, you can still benefit from bodybuilding and strength training regularly. Increasing your muscle mass will help to reduce the stress and impact on your joints and bones. Consider the amount of stress that each step you take while running can have on your knees. Stronger leg muscles can help take some of the strain off your joints by absorbing the majority of the impact. Emotional and mental health are improved by muscle building.

Again, muscles may not be solely responsible for improving your mental and emotional health, but resistance training can help support a healthier state of mind. When you exercise, your brain releases endorphins, which are feel-good hormones. These are also known as the "happy hormones." They are in charge of making you feel like you've accomplished something and putting you in a good mood. They are frequently described as having the ability to provide people with a natural high.

Muscles Increase Your Lifespan

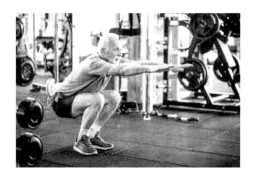

Finally, having a lean mean fighting machine for a body is likely to increase your lifespan. For starters, we've already discussed how having less body fat and more muscle mass makes you less likely to contract certain harmful diseases and illnesses. That alone can significantly increase your chances of living a longer life. However, having better mental and emotional health as a result of regular exercise can help you live longer. This mental and emotional boost can help you relieve stress, which is one of the leading causes of death in the medical world. Consistent exercise also strengthens your immune system, making you more resistant to stress.

That's all there is to it. These are just a few of the most important advantages of devoting more time and effort to body sculpting. Of course, you're probably eager to get started by now, but you need to slow down a little. Remember that you must first devise a strategy. To improve your physical fitness, you must follow a structured and methodical approach. The first step is to understand how your body works and the science behind biomechanics, metabolism, catabolism, and other muscle-building concepts.

Chapter One

Muscle Building Fundamentals

We must first discuss the biological aspects of muscle building before moving on to the practical aspects. Don't be concerned. This isn't going to be some complicated scientific debate about physiology and biomechanics. You do not need to be a medical doctor or have a biology specialization to understand everything that will be discussed here. We'll keep things as simple as possible. Again, this is a book that is intended for anyone to read and comprehend. You won't have to worry about coming across ideas or concepts that you won't understand or apply to your own life.

In this chapter, we'll look more closely at what happens in your body when you exercise and try to gain muscle. When you perform a bicep curl, your muscles do not magically grow slightly with each repetition. That is not how muscle development works. It's a lot more complicated greater than that by the end of this chapter, you'll have a better understanding of how your muscles gain mass and what you can do to stimulate that process.

Consider the information in this first chapter to be a prerequisite for everything you'll learn in the rest of the book.

This will serve as the foundation for all of the knowledge you will acquire, and it is critical to your journey toward achieving the body of your dreams. This chapter will cover topics such as clean and dirty bulking, hypertrophy, rest and recovery, range of motion, strength imbalance, and others. This chapter lays the groundwork and blueprint for the future version of yourself.

How do Muscles Develop?
The Hypertrophy Science

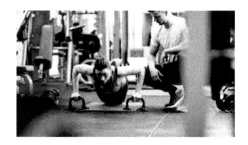

You already know that going to the gym, lifting weights, and eating protein can help you bulk up and gain muscle. You probably know this because of your exposure to popular media, or you may have some gym-going friends. And, yes, these activities can certainly help with muscle growth. But how exactly?

That's what we'll try to explain in the simplest terms we can right now. Hypertrophy refers to the process of building muscle. This is the process of increasing and growing muscle cells in your body, according to science. There are two types of hypertrophies that you should be aware of, especially when developing your strength and training program.

The first is myofibrillar hypertrophy. This is concerned with the expansion of the body parts involved in muscle contraction. Sarcoplasmic hypertrophy is another condition.

This is an increase in the ability of your muscles to store glycogen. These two hypertrophy classifications may not seem important to the average person. However, if you're serious about honing your skills, you'll need to pay closer attention. Myofibrillar hypertrophy is the process of increasing the strength and speed of your muscles. This means that when you do this type of muscle building, your movements will be more explosive. Sarcoplasmic hypertrophy, on the other hand, is associated with long-term efforts and endurance. This type of training allows you to move for extended periods.

Now, the question is, how exactly does hypertrophy work? It's just a matter of breaking to build. You must break down your muscle fibers to make room for new fibers to grow and add to your mass. It's as simple as that. Muscle fibers will break and become damaged whenever you perform a movement that stresses them at a certain frequency. This is why you may feel sore for a day or two after a heavy lifting session. Your soreness is caused by damaged muscle fibers in your body. Now that these fibers have been broken, you must replace them to maximize recovery by loading up on protein. Proteins are made up of amino acids, which play an important role in muscle development and recovery. Protein molecules enter your bloodstream and travel to areas of your body where muscle fibers are broken when you consume them. They will then fill in the gaps and contribute to your body's overall mass.

This may all seem theoretical to you, so let's try to paint a clearer picture of what happens in your body when you try to build muscle. Consider performing a few bench press repetitions. This is a movement that requires you to use your pecs, triceps, and front shoulders. The more reps you do at a difficult weight, the more you are effectively stressing these muscles to the point of mechanical damage and metabolic fatigue. This means that your muscles are deteriorating and losing the energy required to sustain this movement for an extended period. This is why, as you complete more reps on the bench press, the reps become increasingly difficult.

Certain movements become easier to perform as the muscles grow larger and stronger over time. This is why the concept of progressive overload is critical in muscle building.

To return to the bench press example, suppose you begin by performing five sets of five reps of the bench press at 135 lbs. three times per week. It may feel very difficult for you after the first couple of sessions. But it gets easier each time.

This is because your muscles are adapting to the movement and growth. If you stick to this workout routine, your muscles will be less likely to break and hypertrophy. This is why it's best to gradually increase the intensity or volume of your workouts over time. After a few weeks of lifting 135 lbs. with a 5x5 rep scheme, you can experiment with increasing the load or the number of reps. You might be able to do 145 lbs. with the same rep scheme, or you could keep the load and add another set to each session. This way, you are constantly stimulating and challenging your muscles to the point of fibril breakage.

Hypertrophy Approaches
Calorie Consumption and Muscle Growth

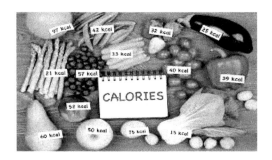

We've discussed how hypertrophy is essentially a breaking-to-build process. You have to break down your muscle fibers to build them up. While there is no other natural way to build muscle than through hypertrophy, the break-to-build method has many variations. In particular, we will concentrate on two main methods in this book. There are two types of bulk: slow and lean bulk and overloaded dirty bulk. Before we get into the differences between these two methods of bulking up, you should familiarize yourself with the roles that calories play.

When you think of calories in the fitness industry, you might think of them as substances you should avoid because they will make you fat. However, most people are unaware that calories in and of themselves are not fattening. Every food contains a certain number of calories, and these calories are made up of vital nutrients that your body requires to function. We previously discussed how protein is an essential component of the hypertrophy process. Every gram of protein you consume contains approximately four calories. Your body would not be able to function without calories. You wouldn't be able to make it.

Whether you realize it or not, your body consumes calories every second you are alive. You may be aware that strenuous movements such as running, jumping, and heavy lifting can burn a significant number of calories. What you may not realize is that even when you're lying down, you're still burning calories. Even when you sleep, you are burning calories. This is because your calories are converted into glucose, which your body uses as fuel to function properly. Every time your heart beats, energy is expended.

Your lungs require energy every time they contract and expand. Whenever your intestines process and digest food, they need calories. This means that the food you eat is converted into energy, which is responsible for your organs functioning properly.

However, calories are frequently demonized in the fitness industry because many people overeat to the point where they consume more calories than they burn. We all have different caloric needs based on our body composition and the activities we engage in daily person with a larger build who works as a hauler will need more calories per day than a slender person who works at a desk. In terms of muscle-building training, you will need a certain number of calories to maintain your daily output. If you don't consume enough calories, especially protein, you endanger the entire hypertrophic process. This is because you are not providing enough protein to your muscles to aid in the building process. Later in the book, we'll go over calories and general nutrition in greater depth. This is a topic that deserves its chapter, and numerous other details must be addressed.

Clean vs. Dirty Bulk

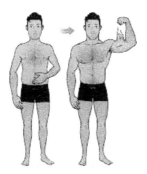

When planning your diet and training program, you should be familiar with two concepts: caloric deficits and caloric surpluses. A caloric deficit occurs when you consume fewer calories than your body requires to function daily. This can also mean that sore and broken-down muscle fibers will take longer to recover. When you consume more calories than you use, you have a caloric surplus. This ensures that your body gets the calories it needs to function, but it can also lead to weight gain and the development of fatty tissues if done excessively.

Given this, bodybuilders will typically take one of two approaches to muscle building: clean bulking or dirty bulking. A clean bulk occurs when someone engages in strenuous strength training and consumes just about the right number of calories, hovering just above the line in terms of how much they burn off each day. So, if you calculate that you burn approximately 3000-3500 calories per day, that is also the number of calories you consume when on a clean bulk.

The benefits of this method include the ability to ensure that you are never overeating. You are still undergoing hypertrophy while limiting fat development. However, with this type of dieting method, you may not be eating as much as you should be. Calorie counting isn't a precise science.

This is why, with this approach to hypertrophy, progress may appear to be slow and minimal. Then there's the soiled bulk. This occurs when you engage in intense strength and resistance training and consume significantly more calories than you are aware of burning each day.

Clean bulking entails sticking to your caloric output every day. Dirty bulking have you consistently crossed that line? Some people may benefit from this if they want clearer and more immediate results from their hypertrophy.

Should You Do Cardio While Muscle Building?

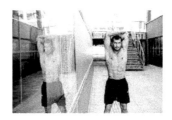

There's a reason why the fitness community is still divided on the subject to this day. There is no simple solution that applies to everyone. Again, it will always be case by case, depending on a person's physiological makeup and goals. Don't be concerned. This is not an excuse. In general, the answer to the question "Should you do cardio while building muscle?" is always yes. Cardiovascular exercises are beneficial to the heart and can benefit everyone. However, that is not the appropriate question to pose. Rather, the correct question is how much cardio should you do when trying to build muscle. However, before you can answer that question, you must first address two others. What body type do you have, and what are your goals?

Taking Care of Your Body Type

Are you naturally thinning and seem to stay that way no matter how much you eat? Do you already have a large build, but it's mostly flab? Are you the type of person who appears to gain muscle quickly? All of these are questions you should ask yourself to determine your body type. In the following chapter, we will delve deeper into the science of body types. But for now, you should know that the more fat you have in your body, the more cardio you will need to do. Building muscle through strength and resistance training can, of course, aid in fat loss.

You can, however, supplement your fat loss efforts by engaging in more cardiovascular activities such as running or jumping rope.

Meeting Your Objectives

Another important factor to consider is the goals you have set for yourself. As a general rule, the leaner and more defined your muscles appear, the more cardio you may need to do than the average bodybuilder. However, if you're more concerned with bulk and less concerned with the definition, you shouldn't be concerned with cardio at all.

In conclusion

This is why, when it comes to answering this question, the fitness community remains divided. No single answer is appropriate for all bodybuilders. It all depends on your interpretation of your situation and goals. Finally, the best you can do is identify the best theoretical framework to follow and adopt it for yourself. If you get the desired results, that's fantastic. If you don't feel like you're making progress over time, don't be afraid to start over.

The Value of Sleep and Recovery

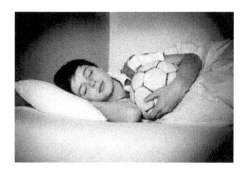

We won't go into detail about this concept in this first chapter because it's far too complex and deserves its water. However, it is still critical to emphasize the importance of incorporating sleep and recovery into your muscle-building strategy. There will be plenty of people who will create the most detailed diet plans and comprehensive training programs for you to follow, which is a good thing. However, it is also critical that you develop a good sleep and recovery plan for yourself. Good sleep is what gives you the energy to keep up with your strenuous workouts every day. Your recovery time is also critical because this is where the "build" aspect of the break-to-build process occurs.

You are breaking your muscles by spending time at the gym training. Your body is rebuilding itself during the time you spend recovering. Again, this is something you will be briefed on in greater detail in a later chapter. But for now, it's important to understand that sleep and recovery are essential components of the muscle-building process.

Chapter Two

Understanding Your Body Type

Not everyone is wired in the same way. This is why the concept of bodybuilding is far more complicated than most people believe. A training program that works for one person may not necessarily work for another. You and a friend may share the same personal trainer and training routine, but you may not achieve the same results. You may be doing the same things, but your bodies may be reacting differently. This chapter will provide you with more information about the various Body types and their distinctions

It is critical that you fully comprehend your body type because it is the most important tool for achieving peak fitness. Not a barbell is the most important tool. This is not a dumbbell. This isn't a squat rack. It's your own body. This is why you should spend some time getting to know your body's ins and outs and figure out your body type Once you understand your body type, you will be able to plan your strategy for achieving your fitness goals and objectives.

The 3 Major Body Types

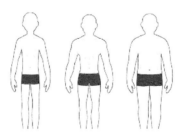

In bodybuilding, there are three distinct body types that most people fall into. These body types can have a significant impact on how your body responds to training stimuli, nutrition, recovery, and other factors involved in muscle building. Given that, learning the ins and outs of your body type will help you understand what you need to do to succeed.

It was mentioned that there are three distinct body types that we will be discussing here; however, it is important to note that you are not always limited to one category. People may begin with one body type when they are younger and then gradually transition to another as they get older. Genetics, lifestyle, physical activity, health history, and other factors all play a role in determining your body type. With that out of the way, let's dive right into the differences between being an ectomorph, endomorph, or mesomorph.

Ectomorph

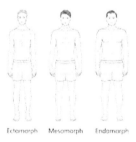

Ectomorph   Mesomorph   Endomorph

The ectomorph is the first body type to be discussed here. This is the type of person who finds it difficult to gain weight despite feeling full after eating. The ectomorph has a difficult time gaining fat or muscle and is often referred to as a hard gainer. Ectomorphs will need to consume a lot of leaner protein (sometimes with the help of supplements) to result when trying to build muscles. Furthermore, ectomorphs progress more slowly than other body types when it comes to building strength. They are also prone to losing weight much faster than others when they do not eat enough.

Ectomorphs struggle with weight gain primarily due to their fast metabolism. They have bodies that are so efficient at processing carbohydrates and converting them into fuel for energy that none of them are stored as fats in the body. Ectomorphs should limit their cardiovascular activity as much as possible to void wasting calories that could jeopardize their muscle-building efforts.

What Is the Appearance of an Ectomorph?

An ectomorph who does not exercise or do any type of resistance training will typically have the build of a marathon runner. They may have visible abs as a result of having no belly fat rather than from core exercises. Ectomorphs can have a little fat around the body at times, but the fat is still contained in a relatively small frame.

The Ectomorph's Dos and Don'ts

The first thing you should remember as an ectomorph is to avoid using the treadmill as much as possible. There's no reason for you to do cardio. Cardio is typically used as a fat-burning tool in a bodybuilding program to highlight muscle definition.

However, because you are an ectomorph, your body is already doing a good job of fat-burning on its own. When you do cardio, you risk burning more calories than you want, and your muscles end up being broken down and converted into energy as a result.

Compound movements should make up the vast majority of your training regimen. These are movements that are intended to recruit various muscle groups to perform a given task accurately and safely. Look for high volumes in terms of rep schemes as well. Given your body type, this is the best way for you to gradually increase your strength.

Finally, ensure that you are eating a high-calorie diet. Again, your body type allows for rapid digestion and calorie burning. This means that you must constantly replenish your energy stores so that your body does not break your muscles. To bulk up, consume a lot of healthy complex carbs and lean protein. Healthy fat, such as that found in olive oil or nuts, can also help your body process nutrients more efficiently. Fats also have more calories per gram than the other two macronutrients. Also, don't be afraid to use supplements to ensure that you're getting all of the nutrients you need to keep up with your workouts.

Endomorph

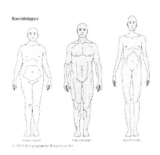

An endomorph is a person who excels at retaining fuel storage. They have more fat and muscle mass concentrated on the lower extremities of the body. Endomorphs, according to many trainers and experts, have the most difficult time managing their weight and developing overall fitness. Gaining weight will be a relatively simple process for you if you are an endomorph. Losing weight and reducing fat, on the other hand, will be more difficult for you than for others.

You will most likely have a wider torso and legs. It's simple to gain muscle, but it's difficult to gain LEAN muscle. That means that while you may be building muscle through caloric surpluses, you're also likely to be getting fatter.

Of course, this does not mean that you will never be able to achieve a lean and trim body. Many endomorphs have chiseled physiques as a result of their hard work and strict adherence to their fitness regimens. You just need to make sure you put in the effort at the gym and in the kitchen with your diet. It is very easy for you to gain strength, but losing fat while maintaining that strength may prove difficult.

What Is the Appearance of an Endomorph?
If you are an endomorph, you are most likely to have a stocky or blocky build. You may have a wider rib cage than most people, and your hips may be as wide as, if not wider than, your collarbones. You may also have thicker joints and flabbier limbs than the average person. Endomorphs can still have muscle definition, but they will most likely be accompanied by fat lumps. The most visible endomorphs in sports are American football players, sumo wrestlers, and Olympic weightlifters.

The Endomorph's Dos and Don'ts

The first thing you may be doing incorrectly as an endomorph is spending hours on a treadmill or elliptical machine. Sure, it may seem like a good idea to devote more time to cardio work because you aren't necessarily built lean, but this isn't an efficient use of your time, especially if you want to build muscle. Instead of doing slow steady-state cardiovascular work, try bursts or intervals of high-intensity training. You get all of the benefits of fat burning while exercising, as well as revving up your metabolism for when you're not exercising. Instead of running at a steady pace on a treadmill for 30 minutes, try alternating between 15-minute intervals of 30-second sprints and 30-second walks.

Lifting heavier loads is another thing you should do. You may believe that because you are stockier, you should prioritize fat loss over muscle building. You can, however, use muscle building as a tool to help you burn fat more effectively.

The best way to accomplish this is to lift heavy weights for low to moderate reps with short rest periods in between sets.

Limit your carbohydrate intake as much as possible in your diet. As a result, your body will be forced to use stored fat as fuel. Consume plenty of lean protein and fiber. This is simply to ensure that your muscles are constantly fed while your body is burning stored fat for fuel. This means you should avoid foods like bread and rice.

Increase your consumption of green vegetables as a source of carbohydrates.

Mesomorph

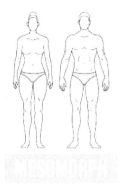

When it comes to body types for bodybuilding, if you are a mesomorph, you should consider yourself lucky. You have the body type that is best suited for gaining lean muscle without gaining too much fat. It will be easier for you to achieve your desired athletic physique than it will be for an endomorph who is stocky or a skinny ectomorph.

Many people all over the world appear to be athletes despite having poor nutrition and exercise regimens. These are the people who are most likely to be classified as mesomorphs. It's important to remember, however, that body types aren't always fixed. Just because you were a mesomorph in your teens and early twenties doesn't mean you'll always be one. Often, as you get older, your metabolism slows down, making it more difficult to keep the fat off. This is why, to stay healthy and fit, mesomorphs must continue to incorporate healthy training and nutrition habits into their daily lives. When competing against the other two body types, being a mesomorph gives you a physiological advantage. But that doesn't mean you shouldn't put in the time and effort required to achieve the body you desire.

How Does a Mesomorph Appear?

Finally, a mesomorph is someone who appears to spend a significant amount of time at the gym even when this is not the case. Furthermore, mesomorphs tend to gain muscle mass quickly. They also find it much easier to gain strength and explosiveness in a short period.

You have broad shoulders and a strong-looking chest, just like an endomorph. You will, however, be much trimmer around the waist than the endomorph. You're less likely to gain belly fat. You are also more likely to have sculpted legs. Especially the quadriceps and calves.

The Mesomorph's Dos and Don'ts

Again, because mesomorphs are typically blessed with good genetics, they are likely to become complacent with their diet and training. This may not appear to be a problem at first. However, over a long period, this

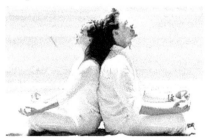

can be extremely harmful. As a result, mesomorphs must set more measurable and tangible goals for themselves. They will be more motivated to exercise if they are chasing real goals.

Also, as much as possible, incorporate regular progression into your workouts. Again, you have good genes, and you will most likely develop your strength much faster than the other two body types. This means that you must constantly increase the difficulty of your workouts so that your progress does not plateau. If you make your workouts difficult, you are introducing new stimuli every time you train. Incorporate more explosive movements into your training routine as well. Focus on functional movements such as box jumps, sprints, pull-ups, and other training tools that translate to daily function.

Last Thoughts

There's no need to be discouraged because of your body's genetic makeup, no matter what body type you have. You may believe that others will have an advantage because they have a certain body type. But the struggle continues. After all, no one achieves their ideal body without putting in the effort. It makes no difference whether you are an ectomorph, endomorph, or mesomorph. You won't get anywhere if you're lazy and unmotivated.

Finally, having better tools to help you succeed is beneficial. All of these tools, however, are useless unless you use them.

It is advantageous to have an ideal body type. However, not having an ideal body type should not be a deterrent. Remember that the journey you're about to embark on is entirely yours and yours alone. It makes no difference if others are making faster progress than you. You are the only one who needs to be focused on here. You may be aware that your body type has advantages or disadvantages in comparison to others.

That is not the point, the goal of this entire chapter is to show you how your body reacts to various stimuli so that you can design the best training plan for your specific needs.

It's all too easy to become discouraged when you look at your body and realize you don't have the natural body type you desire. However, that is not a valid reason for you to avoid doing the work. Learning more about your body type should serve as motivation to work even harder. The more knowledgeable you are about your body's physiological makeup, the better position you will be in to achieve your desired body.

Chapter Three

Nutrition

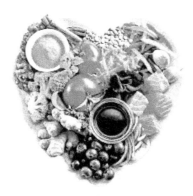

Building the perfect body isn't just about what you do in the gym, contrary to popular belief. You can do all the bicep curls and back squats you want. However, if you have poor eating habits, you will never fully realize your body's potential. A bad diet cannot be outrun, both literally and metaphorically. It's as simple as that. As a result, this section of the book will concentrate on the work you do in the kitchen rather than in the gym. You 'realize that everything you put in your mouth can do far more for your body than anything you can do with a barbell or weights.

This is a fairly consistent theme throughout the book, but there isn't any one way to go about dieting. Diets can have varying effects on different people. You saw a hint of it earlier when we discussed the various body types and how these people have different needs in terms of training and nutrition. This chapter will not necessarily advocate for one diet over another. Don't count on it.

Rather, you can expect to gain a more in-depth understanding of fundamental nutrition principles, allowing you to determine what type of diet would best suit your body type and training regimen.

In this chapter, we'll go over the fundamentals of macronutrients and why you should care about them. We'll also delve deeper into the concepts of metabolism and calories, as well as how you can create your metabolic plan based on your lifestyle and body type. You will also be given examples of healthy food items and meals that you should include in your diet. Finally, you will be given concrete tips and tricks to help you make the most of your diet as you work toward your ideal body.

The Nutritional Contribution to Muscle Growth

It's time for a hot take: going to the gym is a waste of time if you're going to eat a lot of crappy food for every meal. You probably already know from your childhood lessons that you need to eat a well-balanced diet to stay healthy. This is why, as a child, you were probably forced to eat vegetables even though all you wanted to eat was hotdogs and cereal. Hopefully, you've grown out of that phase and developed a more refined palate. Of course, some adults eat more vegetables now than they did when they were younger. But how much is the right amount? Should you consume more meat? Isn't it true that eating meat is bad for you? Are all fats harmful? So, why do some people believe that there are good fats?

These are all valid concerns that you may have.
Nutrition is a complicated game, which is why many people are afraid to start a new diet. However, the more you learn about nutrition and its

fundamental principles, the simpler and clearer everything becomes. This is especially true if you are the type of person who is concerned with the appearance and functionality of your body And if you're reading this book, there's a good chance you are that type of person.

Building the ideal body is not a feat that can be accomplished solely through hard training. Again, this is a break-to-build process, and the training you do in the gym is just the beginning.

The food you consume is responsible for the development of your physique. For one thing, food will provide you with the energy and strength to complete your workouts. Furthermore, food is in charge of strengthening your muscles and joints to the point where they improve your build and overall physique.

That is precisely how you should think about your relationship with food. You will never be able to perform well in the gym if you do not eat properly. You also won't be able to grow your muscles if you don't feed them properly. Nutrition plays two roles in muscle building. It affects both your performance and the overall appearance of your body. If you obsess over the amount of weight you pull and the number of reps you perform, you should do the same with your food. You must obsess over the number of calories you consume and the amount of protein you consume. These are all minor details that can add up to a significant impact and success for your body over time.

Protein's Importance

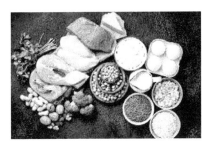

Bodybuilders and athletes, as you are probably aware, rely heavily on protein. But, if you're new to nutrition, you might not realize that protein is only one of three macronutrients you should be including in your diet.

Yes, protein is an essential building block for nourishing your muscles and strengthening your joints. However, you can't live solely on protein. You must understand the relationship that protein has with your body as well as the other macronutrients. This way, you can take a more comprehensive approach to understand your nutrition and creating a plan for yourself.

Identifying the Three Macronutrients

If you recall all of your previous nutrition lessons, you may recall that each food item may be high in a specific nutrient. You may also recall that each nutrient has a distinct benefit for your body. For example, you may have heard that carrots are high in Vitamin A. This meant that your vision would improve. You may also be aware that oranges are high in Vitamin C. This means they can assist you in strengthening your immune system. Now is a good time to become acquainted with all of these nutrients and the foods that contain them.

However, for muscle building, there are only three nutrients that you should pay close attention to. They are known as macronutrients, and they consist of carbohydrates, fat, and protein.

In this nutrition segment, you will learn about the different macronutrient values and the roles they play in your quest to build muscle. It's not just about consuming as much protein as possible. You don't want to be a jerk. You will be in a better position to have a truly more well-balanced diet once you have a better understanding of all three macronutrients... the same one that your grade school teachers and parents tried to teach you about when you were younger.

Carbohydrates

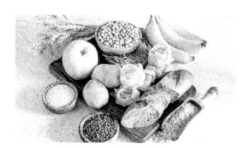

Carbohydrates, or carbs for short, are the first macronutrient you should be aware of. Carbohydrates frequently get a bad rap in the fitness community because they are closely associated with foods such as donuts or pizza. Naturally, if you consume large quantities of those specific foods, you will gain weight. While these high-carb foods may be unhealthy, carbs in and of themselves are not.

Carbohydrates contain only four calories per gram. This is significantly fewer calories per gram than fat. However, the issue with carbohydrates for muscle building isn't just how many calories they contain. It is more about how your body processes those calories internally. Carbohydrates are readily available to fuel sources for your body. When your body detects carbs in your system, it immediately begins the process of converting those carbs to glucose. This glucose will be your fuel as you run, jump, lift, breathe, and do anything else that requires the recruitment of any part of your body. So, if you go to the gym regularly, you'll need carbohydrates to fuel your workouts. Carbohydrate consumption may even provide you with an extra boost during your workouts at times.

Any leftover carbs that aren't used for energy will be converted into stored fat for later use. It's essentially your body's way of preparing itself for when you need a quick source of energy but don't have immediate access to food.

Given this, it is critical that you only consume as many carbohydrates as you require at any given time. This ensures that you are only using the exact amount of carbs that your body requires to sustain the movement and that none of it is converted into stored fat. The precise amount will vary from person to person depending on training intensity, volume, and body type. However, as a general rule of thumb, the number of carbs you should consume should be roughly twice the number of grams of protein you consume. If you are an endomorph who quickly gains weight,

You might want to be more conservative with this approach and limit your carbohydrate intake to 1x-1.5x your protein consumption.

The discussion of carbs does not end there. You should also be aware that there are two types of Simple and complex carbohydrates Simple carbohydrates are quick-acting sources. They are the carbohydrates required to complete the task quickly and effectively They're widely available and quickly depleted. Then there are the complex carbohydrates. Complex carbs take longer to digest, but they provide a more sustained steady stream of energy to the body. Consider simple carbohydrates to be energy for workouts such as short sprints, whereas complex carbohydrates are more beneficial for marathons. We'll go over specific examples of both types of carbs later.

Fat

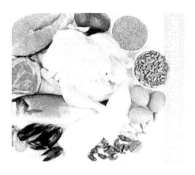

The following item on the agenda is fat. Contrary to popular belief, eating fat does not automatically lead to obesity. Fat, like carbs, has gotten a bad rap in the fitness community due to its name and the number of calories it contains per gram. For example, some people believe that the fat they have around their bellies, arms, or thighs is due to the fat they consume from oil or meat. But that's not how fat works, and it's also not how your body processes fat. Just because you eat the fatty part of a steak doesn't mean it will translate into belly fat.

Fat is a very powerful micronutrient that aids your body in absorbing and processing all of the other nutrients it requires to function properly. In a way, they are critical to the muscle-building process because they help your muscles absorb more protein and recover more quickly from strenuous workouts. Fat is also responsible for improving your body's immune system, and it can be used as an energy source when your body runs out of carbohydrates.

Like carbohydrates, not all fatty foods are created equal. Fat is classified into two types: saturated and unsaturated.

Essentially, the two can be distinguished based on how they appear at room temperature. Unsaturated fats typically take on a liquid form at room temperature, whereas saturated fats remain solid. When incorporating fats into your diet, you should aim to consume as many unsaturated fats as possible. These are the facts that are responsible for all of your body's positive health effects on its internal processes. Saturated fat-rich diets, on the other hand, are frequently linked to diseases such as stroke, cardiac disease, and hypertension.

Protein

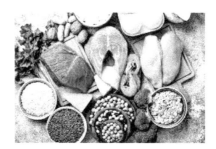

Finally, protein is every bodybuilder's favorite macronutrient. Proteins are made up of various types of amino acids. They are frequently referred to as the foundation of any muscle tissue. Consider a large, sturdy house with sturdy walls and a protective roof. That house would not be as strong and sturdy without the cement blocks that were used to fortify it. Protein is essentially the building block of your body. This is why protein is so popular in fitness, particularly for muscle and strength-building.

So, what are some of the practical advantages of protein? First and foremost, it is necessary to increase strength and mass. The more protein you put into your muscles, the stronger and bigger they will become. This is why lifting a bunch of weights at the gym but not eating enough protein to supplement it is completely pointless. All of your efforts will be for naught. Protein is also responsible for facilitating your body's recovery process after strenuous workouts. It can help repair any breaks in your muscle tissues and joints, allowing you to return stronger and fitter than before you started working out. Protein is also lower in calories than fat. Protein, like carbohydrates, contains only four calories per gram.

However, it is critical that you do not consume more protein than is necessary. If you eat a lot of protein but don't do the resistance training that goes along with it, all of that protein will be converted to fat. Strength training is required to create those breaks in your muscle fibers where protein can swim to and repair. If these breaks do not exist, the protein you consume will be processed and converted into stored fat.

Metabolism and Calories

We discussed these two ideas in the first chapter of this book. Now we're going to change things up by approaching the ideas in this segment in a more practical and applicable manner.

Before we do that, let's go over some basics. Any food that you consume has a caloric value. A medium-sized egg, for example, can contain up to 70 calories, while a cup of rice can contain up to 250 calories. Food contains calories because it contains nutrients that feed and nourish your body. Your body processes the calories in your food and uses them as fuel for daily functions. If you consume calories that exceed the amount of energy you expend, you are in a caloric surplus. If you do not consume enough calories, you will experience a caloric deficit.

How do you know how many calories your body is burning? Everything is determined by a process known as metabolism. This is your body's ability to convert the calories you consume into energy. The greater your body's metabolism, the more calories you burn at any given time. If you have a slower metabolism, the opposite is true. Given that, if you have a higher metabolism, you will burn more calories per day than someone with a lower metabolism, even if you eat the same amount of food. If your body has more calories than it needs, you are more likely to gain weight over time. If you consume fewer calories than you expend, you will lose weight.

But how exactly do calories affect your weight gain? To put it another way, one pound of fat equals approximately 3,500 calories. So, if your total caloric deficit over a week is 3,500 calories, you will be one pound lighter than the previous week. Instead, if you have a 3,500-calorie surplus, you will gain a pound of fat in a week. It gets a little more complicated when it comes to muscles. A single pound of muscle contains only 700 calories. However, eating 700 calories will not result in you gaining a pound of muscle. It is estimated that you will gain a pound of muscle, you must consume approximately 2700 - 3000 calories from lean protein.

Calculating Your Base Metabolic Rate

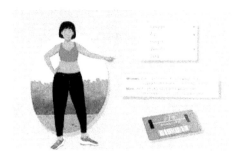

With all of the nutrition knowledge that has been discussed thus far, you may be feeling a little overwhelmed. Don't worry. Finally, the only thing you need to know about calories and metabolism is that it's a game of advantages and disadvantages. The more calories you consume at the end of the day, the more weight you gain, and vice versa. Furthermore, the higher your body's metabolism, the more calories you can burn in a day. Great. So, now that that's out of the way, you should get to work calculating how many calories you burn in a day. Sure, there are smartwatches and fitness trackers that can give you an estimate of how many calories you burn per day. It also helps to be able to perform these calculations on your own. Not everyone will want to spend money on fitness trackers that aren't guaranteed to provide 100% accurate data in the first place.

Before we get into the specifics of calculating your base metabolic rate, we need to make sure you understand what it is and why it is important.

The thing about your body's metabolism is that it is constantly at work, even when you are not aware of it. You could be sitting in front of your computer or sleeping. Your body is still attempting to turn calories into energy. Breathing, cell regeneration, blood circulation, and digestion are all energy-intensive processes.

Most people will step onto a treadmill and see that they are burning a certain number of calories in a single running session. However, the calories you burn while exercising are not the only calories you burn throughout the day. To maintain itself, your body burns calories at other times of the day. Your base metabolic rate is the rate at which you burn calories when you are not exercising.

It is now critical that you determine your basal metabolic rate so that you know how many calories you should consume to maintain yourself without becoming fat or losing muscle.

Again, if you eat excessively, you may gain weight. If you eat too little, your body will not recover as quickly from workouts and you will struggle to gain lean muscle. calculating for It is as simple as following this no-fuss formula

BMR:

For women,

BMR = 655 + (9.6 kg weight) + (1.8 cm height) - (4.7 years of age)

BMR for men = 66 + (13.7 weight [kg]) + (5 height [cm]) - (6.8 age (in years))

How would this calculation look? Assume you're a 29-year-old man standing 180 cm tall and weighing 85 kg. It is simply a matter of substituting values to calculate your BMR.

BMR = 66 + (1164.5) + (900) - (197.2) = 1,933.3

So, based on these calculations in this example, you would be burning 1,933 calories per day, not including any calories burned from exercise. Again, BMR does not take into account any amount of training you may be doing. If you truly want to know how many calories you burn per day, you must first assess your level of activity. Try to categorize yourself as one of the following:

Sedentary - little to no physical activity (multiply BMR by 1.2)

Lightly active - 1-3 times per week of light exercise (multiply BMR by 1.375)

Moderately active - 3-5 times per week, moderate exercise (BMR multiplied by 1.55)

Very active - 6-7 times per week of hard exercise (multiply BMR).

Extremely active - strenuous exercise 6-7 times per week (or more if your job is physically demanding, such as construction or being an athlete).

Of course, these are only estimates. It's not a precise science. The figures could be skewed due to a variety of factors. Take the results of these computations as a guideline for what you should be aiming for and adjust your training/diet plan accordingly. If you see that the results are good, keep going. If you believe your calculations are incorrect, make the necessary changes.

Caloric Excess or Deficit?

Based on your body type, age, gender, and level of physical activity, you may already have a good idea of how many calories you burn each day. You calculated your base metabolic rate and multiplied it by the amount of physical activity you engage in over the course of a week. It's now up to you to figure out how much you should be feeding yourself. Depending on your relationship with food, you may or may not like what you're about to read here. Eating a lot of food (especially bland healthy food like greens and chicken breast) can be difficult for some people. Cutting out bad foods like sweets and junk food can be an even bigger tragedy for many people. Nobody ever said that getting the body of your dreams would be simple.

In this section, we will delve deeper into the concept of caloric surpluses and caloric deficits. What are the advantages of each, and when are they useful? Finally, it comes down to deciding what your objectives are. If you are an ectomorph or a mesomorph with a slim frame, you should consider having a caloric surplus.

To compensate for your level of physical activity, your body expends a lot of fuel and energy. If you want to build lean muscle, you must feed your body a sufficient amount of healthy lean proteins and complex carbs. You don't want to go into a caloric deficit because it will stymie your body's hypertrophy process. Your approaches to caloric surpluses, on the other hand, should be distinct. If you're an ectomorph, you have a little more wiggle room and a higher margin of error when it comes to how many extra calories you can consume per day without getting fat. If you're a mesomorph, you should exercise extreme caution with your caloric surplus. A general rule of thumb is to not consume more than 500 calories per day to maximize muscle growth while minimizing fat gain.

When it comes to fitness, endomorphs have a much smaller margin for error than mesomorphs and ectomorphs preventing fat accumulation Even if you work out hard at the gym, it's very easy for you to gain weight. While going into a caloric surplus is permissible in some circumstances, it is not required.

Sometimes you'd be better off simply balancing your calories burned and calories consumed. Endomorphs can gain muscle while on a caloric deficit in some cases, as long as they get the majority of their calories from protein.

If you want to go into a caloric surplus, make sure you don't go over 300 extra calories per day and incorporate more cardio into your workouts.

Organizing Your Diet Around the Three Macros

You might be getting frustrated with how theoretical many of these concepts have been so far. You are already aware of the term's calories burned and calories consumed. You've already heard of surpluses and deficits. But how does that knowledge translate into the amount of food you should be eating? To create an effective diet plan for yourself, you must first understand the three macronutrients.

How Should Your Plate Look?

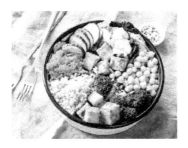

It would be ideal if you paid close attention to every nutrient that enters your body. It is, however, quite impractical. You don't always have to keep track of how much sodium, potassium, or vitamin C you consume with each meal. Looking at your macronutrients is a more practical way of paying attention to your nutrition. Some people prefer to take a more detailed approach to diet, counting the numeric values for calories and macronutrients.

This is an excellent way to immerse yourself in dieting, but it is not required. Sure, there are plenty of fitness and dieting apps to help you track what you're eating and how much of it corresponds to certain nutritional values. All that matters is that you eat enough to feel like you can maintain your physical performance and functionality every day.

If you prefer a more hands-on approach to food tracking, go ahead. Use a traditional food journal or embrace technology by using apps such as MyFitnessPal to help you document your food more thoroughly. However, for many people, a simple eye test would suffice. If you want to build lean muscle while losing fat, try to keep your daily calorie intake at a 40-30-30 ratio. This means that 40% of your daily calories should come from protein sources, while 30% should come from each of the other two macronutrients, fats, and carbs. To put it another way, imagine you have a prescribed diet plan of 2500 daily calories to maintain a healthy caloric surplus.

40% of 2500 equals 1000 calories.
30% of 2500 equals 750 calories.

Given this, you should aim for a macronutrient distribution of 1000 calories of protein, 750 calories of fat, and another 750 calories of carbohydrates.

These values, however, are not absolute. Once again, there are numerous variables at work here. The ideal macro distribution here is largely determined by your objectives. If you're trying to lose weight, higher protein content may be the way to go. So, perhaps a 50-25-25 or 50-30-20 breakdown is appropriate. It all depends on how your body reacts to various dietary formats. You have the freedom and wiggle room to experiment to see what works best for you.

Keep in mind that your body will respond to food intake differently as you progress in your bodybuilding journey. You will almost always encounter plateaus in your fitness journey. If this is the case, the first thing you should do is modify your training. Take note of the progressive overload principle. As you gain strength, you should make your workouts more difficult. If that doesn't work, you may need to change your diet. If you're not gaining muscle as quickly as you used to, you may need to increase your calorie or protein intake. Maybe you're getting a little pudgy and gaining some unwanted fat. This could be a sign that you should reduce your calorie and carbohydrate intake.

Carbohydrate-Rich Food

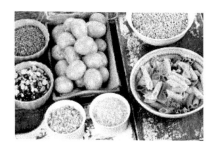

Carbohydrates should ideally account for around 30% of your total caloric intake daily. But not all carbohydrates are created equal. You want to make sure that your carbs come from whole foods that will add nutritional value to your diet. Steel-cut oats have 300 calories, but ice cream has 300 calories. One contains a lot of healthy fiber that will help your digestive system, while the other is high in sugar and will cause insulin spikes. Whole foods also tend to keep you fuller for longer. This means you won't have random cravings for unhealthy junk in the middle of the day. Here are a few examples of the best carbohydrate-rich foods: oats, steel-cut bread made from whole wheat, brown rice or red rice, pasta made from whole wheat, green leafy vegetables (such as lettuce, cabbage, spinach, and kale), tomatoes, red bell peppers, quinoa, potatoes dulcet

Fat-Reducing Food

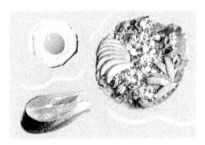

The majority of the time, you just want to avoid foods that contain a lot of trans fats. They are known as bad fats because they hurt a person's cardiac health and overall immune system.

Instead, aim for a high proportion of unsaturated fats and a low proportion of saturated fats. These are fats that contain a high concentration of antioxidants and natural nutrients that aid in the regulation of your body's internal processes.

Unsaturated Fatty Acids

nuts, butter olive oil, seeds of peanuts (pumpkin, sesame, etc.), fatty seafood (salmon, mackerel, etc.), avocados-vegetable oils (canola, corn, sunflower, etc.)

Saturated Fatty Acids

cheese, butter, cream, and meat fat, palm oil coconut oil

Protein-Rich Food

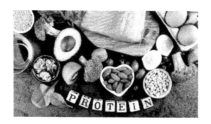

Protein, of course, is a must. You already know that protein serves as the foundation's cement blocks. the musculature of your body So, in any bodybuilding-focused diet, you want to make sure that you are getting enough protein.

A healthy serving of lean protein derived from natural food sources. Most of the time, protein can be obtained from meats such as beef, chicken, pork, and fish. However, if you follow a plant-based diet, you can still get protein. Here are some of the most common food protein sources:

Eggs
milk cheese
chicken spork
turkey beef fish nuts and so on.

Avoid At All Costs These Foods

Discipline is a crucial skill to master when you're a student attempting to achieve your ideal physique Many people suffer from hung up on the discipline aspect that focuses on establishing new routines and habits However, there aren't many. People realize that discipline is also about eliminating bad habits that may impede your progress toward your goals. There could be some foods in your current diet plan that you should avoid. If you truly want to maximize, you must eliminate everything. your efforts in strength and resistance training Here are a few examples: of typical culprits of food items that may keep you from achieving your objectives:

Beverages containing alcohol

As difficult as it may be, you'll have to say goodbye to your favorite beers, whiskeys, tequilas, and vodka cocktails for a while. The unfortunate truth is that alcoholic beverages can impair your body's ability to process the nutrients it requires to survive. This means that when you have alcohol in your bloodstream, the muscles you break from resistance training will not be repaired as efficiently with protein.

Furthermore, when you go out for a night of binge drinking with friends, you consume a lot of unnecessary calories. A single serving of beer can easily contain 150 or even 200 calories. You could choose harder liquors with lower calorie counts, but if you mix them with other ingredients like sweeteners or sodas, it's all for naught. A few beers here and there aren't going to do much harm to your body. Simply try to limit your alcohol consumption as much as possible. If possible, try to eliminate it from your diet.

Sugars, whether refined or added

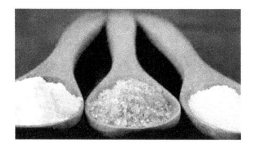

Foods high in refined or added sugars, in general, add very little nutritional value to your body's nutritional intake. Of course, after a hard workout, it's tempting to reward yourself with a delicious donut or a pint of ice cream. However, you would be effectively undoing a large portion of your gym progress. Instead of becoming leaner and gaining muscle, you are simply adding sugar to your body, which is converted into stored body fat and causes you to crash and burn. Instead of rewarding yourself with sugary treats after a workout, try a fruit smoothie or some low-carb protein bars.

At the end of the day, there's no denying that a chocolate bar will taste far superior to a bowl of kale.

But no one ever said dieting would be simple. Limit your intake of sugary sports drinks, sugary coffee beverages, ice cream, cake, donuts, cookies, potato chips, and other similar foods. They're fine for occasional treats, but you shouldn't make it a habit to consume these items regularly.

Deep-fried foods

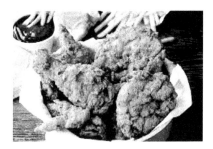

Just because chicken is high in protein doesn't mean you should eat buckets of fried chicken for every meal. Working out at the gym does not give you the right to queue at KFC every day. The truth is that deep-fried foods such as fried chicken and French fries are high in unnecessary calories derived from fat sources such as oil and carb sources such as breading and flour. Furthermore, these deep-fried foods can increase inflammation in your body and slow muscle recovery. Deep-fried foods include fish fingers, chicken nuggets, fried chicken, potato chips, French fries, onion rings, corn dogs, and others.

Bodybuilders' Favorite Supplements

It's now time to talk about supplementation. The first thing you should know about supplementation is that it isn't always necessary to build lean muscle. If you truly commit to eating a clean and healthy diet, you will find success in your fitness goals.

However, for many people, food alone will only get them so far. Some people will find it difficult to consume pounds of lean chicken breast daily to meet protein requirements. This is where supplements come into play. Many people may be hesitant to try supplementation at first due to the negative reputation that these substances may have. Many newcomers may confuse healthy and natural supplements with performance-enhancing drugs such as steroids. These are not the same thing. It is critical to emphasize that using health supplements in moderation is completely safe. Your relationship with supplements should be the same as your relationship with food. You should only consume what your body requires to function optimally. Furthermore, supplements should be viewed as an adjunct to a healthy diet based on food. They should not be used as meal substitutes. You want to get as many of your nutrients as possible from whole foods that are as natural as possible.

Having said that, cycling supplements into your daily dietary rotation can still be beneficial. You simply need to know which supplements to look for, how much of them you require, and what functions they may serve in your training regimen. Here are some of the best supplements for bodybuilding that you should consider purchasing.

Protein from Whey

The first supplement you should purchase is whey protein. This is one of the most popular bodybuilding supplements on the market. This is due to the important bodybuilding effects that protein has on the body. Whey protein is best consumed immediately following a strenuous workout. Preferably within the next 30 minutes. This is because whey is a fast-acting protein that is quickly absorbed by the muscles. Many modern whey protein manufacturers also sell their products in a variety of flavors. Whey protein is typically sold as a powder that can be mixed with other ingredients such as milk, juice, or blended fruits. As a result, whey protein is an excellent post-workout treat or reward.

Protein Casein

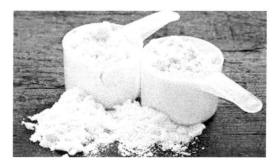

Casein protein is another type of protein supplement that is typically available in powder form. However, it differs from whey protein in the amount of time it takes to process.

To reap the most benefits from whey protein, it must be absorbed into the body within 30 minutes of a hard workout. This is because whey mostly acts quickly. It's not the same with casein. It takes a lot longer.

Before going to bed, most people consume casein protein. This ensures that your body receives a steady supply of protein throughout the night. According to research, the muscle recovery process accelerates during the sleep stage.

Gainers of Weight

If you are an endomorph or a mesomorph who easily gains weight, you may not want to invest in this product. However, if you are an ectomorph who struggles to gain the calories needed to build muscle, you can try weight gainers. These are typically powdered substances that are high in protein, either whey or casein. Aside from that, they are high in carbohydrates, which increases the calories per serving. Again, make sure that this supplement is used in conjunction with a healthy diet that focuses on whole foods. It should not be used to replace a meal.

BCAA (Branched Chain Amino Acids)

Branched-chain amino acids, or BCAA, are made up of three essential acids that are necessary for muscle growth: leucine, isoleucine, and valine. Typically, these acids can be obtained in small amounts from meats, poultry, dairy, and fish. This is essentially a supplement designed for people who do not consume enough protein from whole foods. Again, not everyone will be satisfied with eating chunks of chicken breast or tuna for every meal.

This is where supplements like BCAA come in to help you get the nutrients you need without eating an excessive amount of food.

Creatine

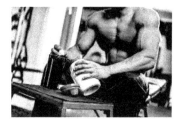

Aside from whey protein, many bodybuilders claim that creatine is their go-to supplement. To begin with, creatine is in charge of transporting all of the water you drink into your muscles. Almost 80% of your muscles are made up of water, and creatine helps keep your muscles hydrated at all times. It is also in charge of providing energy to your muscles so that they are always optimized for peak physical performance when you work out. A regular intake of creatine makes it much easier to gain strength and mass. However, some critics claim that creatine can harm your kidneys or liver because it diverts all of the water you drink away from these organs and instead feeds it to your muscles. This is why it is critical to stay hydrated and drink plenty of water while on a creatine cycle.

Fatty Acids Omega-3

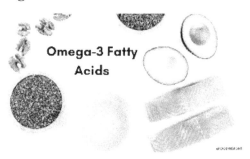

You may be familiar with Omega-3 Fatty Acids as the nutrients found in fish oil gels. This is a supplement that is especially popular among the elderly because it is frequently marketed as a product that relieves joint pains and aches. However, in addition to strengthening your joints, fish oil can aid in the recovery process by reducing inflammation in your muscles. This means that you will be less sore after a hard workout and will be able to put in more effort in the gym the next day.

Caffeine

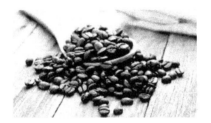

Caffeine, yes. Caffeine is a popular dietary supplement for athletes and people who stay active in general, which many people are unaware of. Caffeine is a favorite among bodybuilders for two reasons. For starters, it boosts the body's metabolism. This means it assists the body in burning more fat while at rest. Another reason caffeine is so popular is that it gives athletes the energy and stamina they need to complete difficult workouts. Caffeine is commonly consumed by marathon runners and endurance athletes before a race.

Caffeine is also commonly consumed by bodybuilders before a heavy lifting session to provide more energy to the muscles.

The Best Nutritional Tips and Tricks

Nutrition is a complex subject. It's understandable if you're feeling a little overwhelmed by everything that's been said thus far. You should not expect to master this in a single day. All of these are very complex concepts that you must gradually integrate into your daily life. It is not something that can be completely absorbed in one sitting. Given this, it may be best to distill all of the information into bite-sized tips and tricks that you can apply in your daily life.

Again, the habits you practice every day will ultimately determine your success. If you apply these simple secrets and tips to your life consistently, you will see results. You won't even have to wait long to feel like you're making progress.

Make Real Food a Priority

Again, it's critical to prioritize real food. And by "real food," we mean food that has undergone as little processing as possible. Avoid overly processed foods like canned meats, bagged chips, and chocolate bars. These aren't real foods, and they won't help you get the body you want. Try to source your meals as much as possible from meats and plants. Make an effort to keep it as clean as possible.

Supplements Should Not Be Feared

Now that you know you should always prioritize real food, let's talk about the importance of supplements. Finally, you should prioritize real food as much as possible. However, there will be times when you simply cannot get the nutrients you require from whole foods alone. This is where supplements can come in handy. For example, you may have reached your daily caloric limit but still require additional protein. A glass of whey protein can help you meet your protein requirements without having to eat a chicken at the end of the day or after a workout.

Consume Plenty of Water

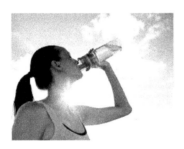

Water, once again, is life. Literally. When you're trying to build muscle, you need to stay hydrated. For starters, your muscles are made of water. Water makes up the majority of your body. You want to ensure that your body is properly hydrated so that it can function properly. Staying hydrated also helps your cells regenerate faster and can aid in muscle recovery. It can also be hazardous to your kidneys if you consume a lot of protein without drinking enough water. Eating too much protein and not enough water can put your kidneys at risk.

Keep Track of Your Food Consumption
You should keep track of what you're eating. You will not be able to maximize your potential and achieve your desired goals if you just wing it.

Sure, some people have enough experience to know how much they should eat without keeping a food journal. This, however, can only be attained through consistent practice and experience. If you're a novice who is just getting started, you should take the time to track what you're eating as accurately as possible. This may appear to be a lot of work, but no one ever said it was going to be easy.

Make a Meal Plan

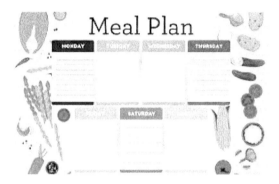

Tracking your meals may appear to be a chore. However, if you plan and prepare your meals, everything becomes much easier and simpler. It only takes one day a week for you to sit down and write down all of the meals you'll be eating over the next seven days. Make a list of everything, including all of your major meals and snacks. This is advantageous for a variety of reasons. For starters, it makes grocery shopping much easier. You will only purchase the ingredients required for your meal plan. Next, you'll find it easier to track your meals and caloric intake if you plan them ahead of time. When you have a plan to follow, it will also help you avoid overeating or undereating throughout the week.

Make Changes Whenever Necessary

The diet plan you begin with is not necessarily the diet plan you will follow for the rest of your life. You must accept that as you get older and fitter, your body will undergo significant changes. This is why it does not always respond the same way to a particular diet plan. It is critical that you constantly evaluate the effectiveness of your diet plan. If you notice that you aren't getting the desired results, be willing to adjust your diet slightly to account for changes in your body or workout routine. If in doubt, eat meat and vegetables.

There will be times when you will be unable to determine what you should be eating. This is especially true when spending nights out with friends or family at restaurants. You may be forced to deviate from your meal plan and order something on the spur of the moment. Don't be concerned. Just keep in mind that lean meats and vegetables are always a good choice. When in doubt, order a salad and some sort of meat. Make sure there is only a small amount of sauce and dressing. This way, even if you're eating outside, you'll know you're still eating healthy.

Sugar vs. Fibrous Carbs

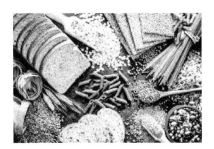

Carbohydrates are not the enemy here. Hopefully, you learned this while reading about macronutrients and the various roles they play in muscle building and overall health. Carbohydrates should always be included in your diet to some extent. When you do eat carbs, however, try to prioritize fibrous carbs over sugary carbs. Choose carbs like wheat and grains because they aid in digestion and nutrient processing. Sugar will only provide you with unsustainable energy and unwanted body fat.

Avoid consuming alcohol.

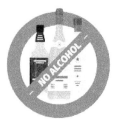

Simply avoid alcohol. Avoid consuming beers and wines because they are high in calories and carbohydrates.

Also, avoid drinking cocktails because they typically contain a lot of unwanted carbs and sugars. Hard liquors may appear to be safe because they are low in calories, but they can seriously impair your body's ability to absorb protein. So, to the best of your ability, try to avoid alcohol. Of course, this does not preclude you from drinking alcohol for the rest of your life. This brings us to our final point...

Take Care of Yourself (Sometimes)

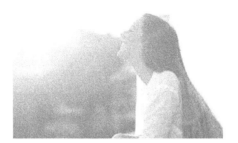

Allow yourself a cheat day now and then. Proceed with caution. If you're not having fun, life isn't worth living. At the end of the day, if you want to be successful, you must learn to enjoy the process. Being strict and constantly disciplining yourself is not enjoyable. Sure, you'll have a lot of success that way. However, never pursue success at the expense of your happiness.

This is why having a cheat day now and then is beneficial. Even as a reward system, this can be excellent practice incorporating into your fitness journey. For example, after a week of strict dieting, you can treat yourself to a scoop of ice cream. To celebrate gaining 5 pounds of muscle, you could go on a one-night drinking binge. Just make sure that these treats are only done on rare occasions. They may not be good for your body, but they are beneficial to your soul.

Last Thoughts

You should be convinced by now that diet plays a significant role in determining how your body will respond to training stimuli. You will never progress as quickly or as efficiently in the gym if you do not supplement your workouts with proper nutrition habits. As tempting as it may be to live on a steady diet of pasta, pizza, burgers, donuts, cookies, ice cream, and beer, you'll need to develop your sense of discipline. To reiterate a point made earlier in this chapter, you can't outrun a bad diet. If you eat junk all the time, your body will never be able to accomplish everything it was designed to do.

It's all too easy to fall into the trap of believing that just because you're working out hard at the gym means you can eat whatever you want. When it comes to designing your diet plan, this is completely the wrong mindset to have. True fitness is a balanced combination of physical activity and nutrition. To achieve optimal health and wellness, you must marry these concepts. Failure to combine a good training regimen with proper nutrition can lead to suboptimal results. It's as simple as that.

Hopefully, this chapter has provided you with useful information and enough motivation to pursue a healthier lifestyle in the kitchen. Not every battle takes place on a racetrack or in a boxing ring. Master the art of proper dieting and nutrition to triumph over unwanted body fat.

Chapter Four

Rest and recuperation

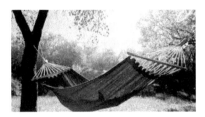

It is not always necessary to work hard. Fitness and nutrition are more than just how hard you work in the gym or how strict your diet is. It also involves how you care for your body in terms of rest and recovery. When you're first starting, it's easy to become addicted to spending all day every day at the gym. This is especially true if you've found a lot of success quickly.

That success can become addictive, to the point where you crave it like a drug. So, because you've found success by working hard at the gym, you believe you can get more of it by spending more time there. In theory, this is possible. In all honesty, you're only human, and you need to rest. You may be doing more harm than good to your body if you do not provide it with the proper care that it requires for you to continue working towards your fitness goals.

This chapter will emphasize the significance of rest, sleep, and general body care. When you first start working out, it can be pretty amazing to see all of the amazing things your body can do. You'll never be able to imagine yourself lifting heavy weights or defining specific muscle groups until you see it happen. Some people spend their entire lives believing that they will never be able to deadlift twice their body weight.

And it's only because they never consider trying. When you see your body performing these incredible feats, it can be tempting to just keep pushing. The problem is that when you don't give yourself time to rest or recover, you end up putting yourself in danger of injury.

There are numerous approaches to keeping your body safe and ready for action in the gym every day. Much of it must be done with specific exercises or habits you can implement, such as mandatory rest days and supplementation. Sleep is another important factor to consider in this situation. Compare working out while running on less than four hours of sleep to working out after feeling fully rested. You will undoubtedly notice a significant difference in your mood.

Aside from giving yourself time to recover, you must also ensure that you protect yourself from injuries through prehab. Always remember that in medicine, prevention is always preferable to cure. Do not wait until you are injured or overworked before beginning soft tissue work or stretching. All of these concepts will be discussed in greater depth throughout this chapter. Again, it isn't just about working out hard and being disciplined in the kitchen all the time. This is the less exciting, less glamorous, and less interesting aspect of fitness. However, there is no denying the significance of these lessons.

The Value of Rest and Recovery

Every successful person you will ever meet will tell you that their success is the result of hard work. No exceptions. You will never achieve your loftiest goals and dreams unless you are willing to work hard and suffer for them. It's all too easy to get caught up in the romanticism of pouring your blood, sweat, and tears into achieving your goals. This is a topic that is frequently sensationalized in today's media. But do you know what part is rarely mentioned? Rest and recuperation Consider a superhero film. You're used to seeing Captain America and the Avengers in action, fighting the world's most heinous villains. You witness them fighting and clawing their way to victory. It's a lot of fun. But what are you missing? Captain America is never seen napping. You never see Batman doing mobility exercises for his muscles. You'll never hear Superman say he needs a day off.

Get up. You are not a superhero, nor do you live in a fantasy world. You may believe your body is capable of great things, which is a good thing. It is always advantageous to be self-assured. However, you must be careful not to overextend yourself here.

True, you are capable of great things. However, you must also take time to rest and recover from greatness.

Every time you go to the gym, you are expected to give it you're all. And as you continue to work out hard, your muscles will break down even more. This has already been covered in previous chapters. You are aware that breaking down your muscles is an important step in the hypertrophy process. When you break down your muscles, you will inevitably become weaker in the short term, only to emerge stronger in the long term. Long-term muscle gains, on the other hand, cannot be obtained solely through hard work in the gym or proper dieting. There is another aspect to this: rest.

Again, after a strenuous training session, you become weaker in the short term. Rest and recovery are in charge of ensuring that you emerge stronger than ever before. When you take time to rest, you allow your muscles to heal from being broken down and beaten up. Your muscles will feel refreshed and ready to move heavier loads at faster speeds once you have recovered through rest. You are also aware that rigorous training can result in a variety of physiological benefits for the human body. Regular exercise can help you improve your blood flow, heart health, respiratory function, digestion, and other areas. However, if you don't give your body enough time to recover between training sessions, these advantages will be lost. Furthermore, engaging in what is known as overtraining can result in performance plateaus and injuries.

What exactly is overtraining?

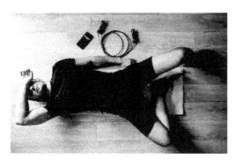

One general principle that can be applied to any aspect of life is that anything done in excess is bad, even if it appears to be beneficial. Of course, this includes training and exercise. Overtraining can be difficult to define because it is a subjective sensation that varies from person to person. A professional runner may be able to run 100 miles per week, whereas the average Joe may only be able to run 20 in the same amount of time. Anything more would be considered overtraining for Joe and just another regular work week for the professional. Everything is relative. This section of the book will provide you with information on how to determine whether you are overtraining or not.

A person's capacity for training can be influenced by a variety of factors. Of course, a lot of it is determined by that person's training history or current level of physical fitness.

However, there are more nuanced factors to consider, such as genetics, age, muscle composition, diet, and so on. In general, an average of 48 to 72 hours of recovery time is required between intense strength training sessions. However, for those who can gradually increase their workload capacity, the length of recovery can be reduced.

Overtraining Symptoms

Now, how would you know if you were overtraining? It would be ideal if you hired a licensed professional to oversee your training so that you wouldn't have to worry about such minor details. If you don't have the luxury of receiving personalized instruction from a professional, you may have to conduct these assessments on your own.

Fortunately for you, the procedure is not too difficult. Finally, the best person to determine whether or not your body is overly stressed is you. When you feel like you're overdoing it at the gym, keep an eye out for the following signs or symptoms of overtraining. These symptoms can be classified as physical or emotional/behavioral.

Physical - enduring muscle

soreness - joint pain - fever - high blood pressure - high heart rate - decreased appetite - unintended weight loss
Emotional/Behavioral irritability, insomnia, depression, anxiety, elevated heart rate, and lack of motivation

Sleep and Its Importance

Many working adults understand that sleep is a valuable resource that few people have the luxury of getting enough of. Too often, people will sacrifice not only the quantity but also the quality of their sleep to be more productive throughout the day. While it may seem more logical to stay up a couple of extra hours at night to get more things done, this can work against your desire to be more productive. Compelling evidence suggests that not getting enough sleep for multiple days in a row can leave you feeling groggy and fatigued throughout the day. As a result, staying focused and motivated to complete specific tasks will be much more difficult.

The same is true for bodybuilding. You might not give much thought to how much time you spend sleeping.

However, you may be unaware that the quantity (and quality) of your sleep has a significant impact on two things: how your muscles repair, recover, and grow, as well as how you perform while training. Essentially, when you sleep, your body enters a deep state of hibernation and self-repair. Your mind switches off and focuses on repairing your body and preparing it for another day of normal activities. You're doing so much more than just sleeping and the brain before falling asleep You're revitalizing your entire body. If you sacrifice your sleep, your muscles will not recover as well as they should. In the end, they won't repair and grow as quickly as you might have hoped.

You can expect suboptimal output and performance whenever you put your body to work as a result of not allowing your body to recover properly due to a lack of sleep. Your muscles were never allowed to repair and rejuvenate properly. As a result, you may still feel sore and tired when you go to the gym. As a result of how tired you are, you will be unable to maximize it. It is critical that you fully comprehend the significance of sleep and how you should incorporate proper sleeping habits into your daily routine.

Knowing Your Sleep Cycles

It's been mentioned a few times that it's not just the amount of sleep that you should be concerned with. It's equally important to pay attention to the quality of your sleep. And before you can fully comprehend what those entail, you must first learn about the various sleep cycles.

When you go to sleep at night, you go through several stages. It's a cycle; a repetitive process in which you alternate between being awake and being immersed in a truly deep sleep until you wake up. Most people can sleep three to five cycles per night, but this varies from person to person.

Stage 1: Awakening

This is usually the stage when you're still slightly awake but gradually falling asleep. You may have noticed this when you find yourself nodding off in the middle of watching TV or reading a book. During this stage, your senses begin to lull you and your heart rate begins to slow.

You're not completely asleep, but you're also not fully awake. This is the time when you are transitioning from a conscious to an unconscious state.

Stage 2: Restful Sleep

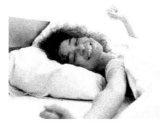

The second stage of sleep involves your brain and muscles winding down. Your brain activity drops significantly, and your muscles relax to the point where they are completely static. You typically enter the light sleep stage 15 to 30 minutes after falling asleep. This is the stage of sleep where you are most easily awakened by external noises or physical cues. As a result, it is known as the light sleep stage.

Deep Sleep (Stage 3)

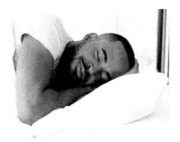

When it comes to bodybuilding and muscle recovery, the deep sleep stage is the one you want to maximize.

Deep sleep is the type of quality sleep that you should always strive for when it comes to repairing your body. This is the stage of sleep in which your brain and muscle activity are so low that they are practically nonexistent. Your heart rate is also most likely at its lowest during this time.

People usually enter a deep sleep stage 45 minutes to an hour after falling asleep. If you are jolted awake from a deep sleep, you will feel groggy and disoriented. You won't be able to detect your surroundings right away, and it will take some time for your mind to adjust to what's going on.

REM (rapid eye movement) is the fourth stage.

Observe your pets, especially your dogs, whenever they go to sleep. Even though their eyes are closed, you may notice that they are moving around quickly. This indicates that they have entered the REM stage of sleep. This is typically the stage of sleep when your brain begins to become active again, causing your eyes to move involuntarily. This is also the stage of sleep during which your dreams occur. The average person's nightly sleeping time is about 25% of REM sleep. Your muscles will become paralyzed during this stage, and your heart rate will gradually increase.

Sleep Deprivation's Negative Effects

Sleep deprivation is something you should always try to avoid if you want to live a healthier and fitter lifestyle.

When you don't get enough sleep at night, you will feel the consequences almost immediately when you wake up. It's one thing to go without sleep now and then.

However, if you do it regularly, you will feel the full force of these negative consequences. It's not just a case of feeling sleepy or tired all day. Other physical, mental, and emotional effects occur when you do not get enough sleep.

As a bodybuilder, you already know that a lack of sleep can stymie muscle growth and recovery. Furthermore, it can result in decreased neurological fitness. This means that when you don't get enough sleep, neurological aspects of fitness like balance, accuracy, timing, and coordination are likely to suffer. Furthermore, sleep deprivation promotes inflammation in the body. This means that swollen muscles will remain swollen for long periods, causing you to feel more sore than necessary.

Other side effects of sleep deprivation include unintended weight fluctuations, mood swings, sugar cravings, a lack of focus, and a weakened immune system.

Working out while sleep-deprived can also make you more prone to injuries.

The Value of "Pre" hub
This entire chapter has been devoted to principles centered on taking care of your body as it is constantly subjected to various stress-inducing environments and conditions.

That is exactly how you should view exercise and dieting. They are stressful situations in which you subject your body to harden and promote self-development. However, it is not healthy to constantly expose yourself to such stressful situations without taking the time to care for yourself.

Remember that the goal here is to complete the entire marathon. It's not going to be an all-out sprint right away. You must ensure that you are thinking in the long term.

It is not always necessary to spend your days lifting heavy weights. You want to work hard, but you don't have to work yourself to muscle failure every time.

This is the quickest way to get to a physical therapy clinic for treatment. When it comes to building the body of your dreams, the last thing you want is to be sidelined for an extended period due to an injury. It's not just about performing exercises safely in the gym. It has more to do with what you do outside of your normal working hours.

This section of the chapter will delve deeper into the concept of mobility and active recovery days. Just because you want to gain muscle doesn't mean your workout should be entirely made up of resistance training exercises. Yes, sleep is important for recovery, but it is not the only thing you can do to ensure that your body is always primed and ready for a hard workout.

Understanding Mobility as an Injury Prevention Tool

If you post a video of yourself foam rolling instead of lifting heavy weights, you won't get as many likes on Instagram. Mobility will never be as flashy or exciting as actual strength and resistance training, but that doesn't diminish its significance. Even though it is not something that everyone enjoys discussing, mobility is an important aspect of fitness that you should incorporate into your routine. So, what exactly is mobility? Many people appear to confuse mobility with flexibility, even though the two are distinct.

Flexibility refers to your muscle's ability to stretch or elongate to a specific length. Mobility, on the other hand, is your body's ability to maintain strength and control while increasing your range of motion. Anyone with enough flexibility can touch their toes without bending their knees. A mobile person, on the other hand, would be able to get into a deep squat without their muscles collapsing or giving way.

Why is mobility so important for a bodybuilder?

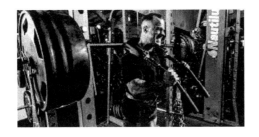

It all comes down to maintaining strength and control while engaging in various explosive movements associated with resistance training. Some people may be able to bench press their body weight. When asked to squat with their hip creases below the knee, these same people will cry out in pain. This may prevent that person from gaining the potential strength gains that come from performing a movement through its entire range of motion. If you only do a half squat because your lack of mobility prevents you from going the full range of motion, you are effectively limiting the movement's potency. You're not engaging as many muscle groups as you should be, and your strength gains will suffer as a result. That is one example of how mobility can benefit you as a bodybuilder.

Another reason why mobility is important is that it protects you from injuries. Athletes who lack proper mobility and push themselves in training far too often end up with tears in their muscles or ligaments. This is because they overtax their bodies, and the stimuli become too much for the body to handle. There's a reason why immobile people experience pain when forced to squat or fully extend a press overhead. Something is wrong with their joints and fascia, preventing them from performing the movement painlessly. Some athletes, whether through adrenaline or sheer willpower, would be able to push through the pain and execute these movements despite their lack of mobility. That pain is meant to act as a safeguard or a limiter. However, once an athlete continues to push past the pain, the body simply gives up.

There are several approaches you could take to improve your mobility. Doing light range-of-motion exercises or dynamic stretches is a common way to increase mobility. These are distinct from static stretches, in which a person holds a stretch for an extended period. These range-of-motion exercises, also known as dynamic stretches, are more kinetic in nature and necessitate constant movement. They are intended to activate muscles and loosen tight spots, particularly those near joints. Another way to improve mobility is to do soft tissue work, such as foam rolling or using a lacrosse ball. Consider your muscles to be made up of tiny little threads known as muscle fibers. When you do resistance training, these threads are stressed and can become entangled. When you exercise, these entangled threads can cause discomfort or a restricted range of motion. You can use tools such as foam rollers, massage guns, or lacrosse balls to help loosen and untangle these muscle fibers and regain a full range of motion. You may also make use of the services.

Being a bodybuilder does not imply that you should only do bodybuilding exercises daily. Your body requires a break from that particular stimulus to recover and grow stronger. Some people even stick to a training regimen for too long, to the point where their bodies become accustomed to it. When this happens, they hit a snag in their progress because their bodies aren't responding to the training stimuli as well as they used to. This is why it's critical to break up your routine with occasional rest days or cross-training. If you have too much energy to go an entire day without doing any kind of exercise, you can have an active recovery day.

Of course, the first option is for you to simply take a day off. Take a day off from the gym and do no exercise at all. It's critical to stick to your diet even on rest days, especially if you're trying to lose fat by going into a caloric deficit. Remember that because you aren't going to the gym these days, you aren't burning as many calories.

Another option is to participate in an active recovery day. This means you make time to do some form of exercise that is less intense and provides a different stimulus than your routine. This can range from shooting hoops in your backyard to a quick yoga session. You can even work on your mobility by simply doing some foam rolling and myofascial release on yourself. The idea is that you are still doing some form of exercise without overstressing your body, just as you would on regular training days.

Track Your Sleep for the Best Sleep and Recovery Habits

Again, getting your eight hours of sleep every night isn't enough. You should also be concerned about the quality of your sleep. This is why you should consider purchasing a sleep tracker. Most modern fitness tracking devices include a built-in heart rate sensor that can aid in the tracking of your sleep cycles at night. These devices will tell you how much time you spend in each stage of a sleep cycle, as well as how many cycles you go through each time you fall asleep. Long-term sleep tracking will also provide you with a better picture of how your performance may be affected by certain sleeping patterns.

Your data may show that getting x amount of sleep per night improves your performance during the day (and during training).

Avoid using blue-light devices late at night.

Unfortunately, we are constantly bombarded with devices that emit blue light. Blue light is emitted by your television, computer monitors, and smartphones. This blue light not only strains your eyes but also prevents you from falling asleep. This blue light sends signals to your brain that mimic the sun's rays. As a result, your brain is tricked into believing that it is still daytime even when you should be falling asleep.

Don't drink coffee after 2 p.m.

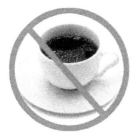

Caffeine is a stimulant that causes your heart rate to increase and provides you with energy. An elevated heart rate and restless energy are two factors that will prevent you from falling asleep.

As a result, it should be common sense to avoid consuming caffeine too close to bedtime. Caffeine's effects last at different times for different people, but a general rule of thumb is that you should never drink coffee after 2 p.m., especially if you want to be in bed by nine or ten p.m.

Take short naps during the day.

Power naps are great as long as they are done correctly. When you are sleep deprived, it can be extremely beneficial to take a few minutes during the day to have a good power nap. Power naps are brief periods of sleep that allow you to recharge your brain in a short period. However, you must exercise extreme caution not to allow these power naps to last too long. Remember when we talked about sleep cycles? If you enter the deep sleep stage, you will feel groggy and disoriented when you wake up from your nap. This is why you should limit your power naps to no more than 30 minutes. Also, avoid taking multiple naps throughout the day. One should suffice.

Make an effort to get up earlier.

One of the main reasons people have difficulty sleeping at night is that they wake up late in the morning. Then, because they woke up late, they have a lot of energy that carries over into the late hours of the night - and the cycle continues indefinitely. You can break the cycle by simply forcing yourself to get up early one morning. Do not press the snooze button. Wake up, get out of bed, and do something useful. Prepare breakfast. Take a walk. Take a hot bath. Do whatever it takes to jolt yourself awake. You will find it much easier to sleep early at night if you also wake up earlier. Again, don't hit the snooze button.

Sleep in a Cool Place

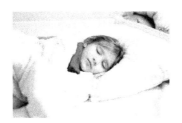

Sleeping in cooler rooms results in better quality sleep, according to research. When you sleep in a cooler environment, you are less likely to be woken up in the middle of the night. Also, sleeping in colder temperatures allows your heart rate to drop more easily. This means your body is better prepared to enter the deep sleep stage of your sleep cycle.

Participate in Cross-Training

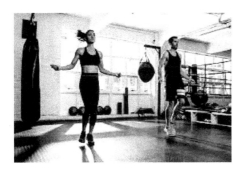

Do some cross-training. Do something unusual for your body. It is critical that you incorporate new stimuli into your training routine so that your body is constantly challenged by new paradigms. Even if you increase the load and volume of your resistance training, your body will eventually reach a plateau. Now and then, go for a run. Attend a yoga class. These are all excellent ways to approach fitness more holistically. It will also keep you from becoming bored by repeating the same routine. Warm-up and cool down properly before and after each training session.

Don't just dive right into a lifting session. If the workout calls for five sets of five reps of deadlifts at 225 pounds, you must ensure that your body is capable of handling that workload. The first thing you should do is warm up by working up a sweat. Perform some dynamic stretches to activate your muscles, improve your range of motion, and raise your heart rate. After that, start with some light deadlift reps and gradually work your way up to your first set at 225 lbs. This is to avoid completely shocking your body into a stressful state. It will also help to prepare your muscles for whatever you are about to put them through.

Then, after a training session, make sure to cool down properly. Perform some mobility exercises such as static stretches or foam rolling. Every day, devote at least 10 minutes to mobility work.

It only takes ten minutes per day to gradually improve your mobility. We've already discussed how mobility can help you improve your performance in the gym and avoid injuries. Simply set aside ten minutes each day to work on a specific muscle group to improve your mobility.

Prioritize areas near major joints, such as your shoulders, hips, knees, and ankles. For example, you could work on your hips today. As a result, you should foam roll your quads, hamstrings, and glutes. The entire procedure will take only ten minutes. The following day, concentrate on your shoulder by massaging your pecs, scapula, lats, and delts.

Again, consistently target different muscle groups, and your mobility will improve over time.

Reduce Your Stress Level in Your Life

Finally, simply reduce the overall level of stress in your life. Don't get too worked up about minor details. If at all possible, try to meditate at different times of the day. Remember to keep things in perspective at all times. Stress has been shown to hurt your body's natural processes. When you go through hard workouts at the gym, you are already stressed.

That should suffice. Any additional stress in your life should be avoided at all costs.

Chapter Five

Muscle Development

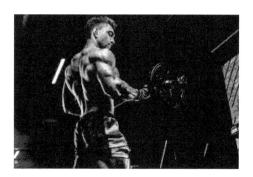

Now it's time to talk about the most exciting aspect of bodybuilding: training. Some people enjoy exercising, while others view it as a chore that must be completed. Regardless of how you feel about exercise in general, it's critical that you have a positive relationship with whatever training regimen you choose for yourself. Nobody should ever be given the same fitness and training regimen. Numerous factors influence what the best training pedagogy should be for you.

However, it should go without saying that the more you enjoy and embrace your training, the more likely you are to stick with it.

That is, at the end of the day, the goal. If you want to see dramatic results, you should strive for consistency through sustained efforts over time. Significant progress cannot be expected in a short period. This is why you must adapt or create a training program tailored to your specific needs.

long-term execution from you to do so, you must first familiarize yourself with the various movements involved in muscle training. You must begin small. This chapter will teach you the fundamentals of training specific muscle groups to promote growth and development. Once you understand how to train specific muscle groups, you will be taught how to combine all of those different exercises to create a cohesive and effective training program for yourself.

It's not enough to know how to get the most out of different exercises to stimulate muscle growth; you also need to know how to do them correctly. You must also learn how to incorporate them into your program. If you perform a specific movement incorrectly, you could cause significant, even irreversible, muscle damage. If you do not properly structure your program, you may be wasting all of your efforts in the gym. It's critical that you understand the nuances of designing a strength training program so you don't end up shooting yourself in the foot.

Before proceeding, you should be proud of yourself for getting this far. Developing the determination to pursue a better body for yourself is something to be proud of. Unfortunately, few people are willing to invest the time, effort, and commitment required to become the best versions of themselves. You are already separating yourself from the pack by doing so. You stand out from the crowd. Now, all that remains is for you to acquire the knowledge required to achieve your objectives most efficiently and effectively possible. After all, none of this knowledge is novel or untested. This is the knowledge that has been passed down through the years by experts and enthusiasts. Muscle building is still a developing science, with breakthroughs and discoveries being made daily. This is why it is critical that you continue to learn by reading books. body pushed to its limits

Isolated vs. Compound Movements

THE COMPOUND LIFTS

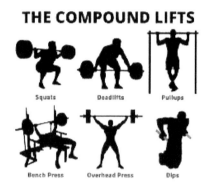

Squats   Deadlifts   Pullups

Bench Press   Overhead Press   Dips

Before we get to the specific movements designed to stimulate muscle building, we must first identify the general classifications of these exercises. Movements in any type of exercise program can be classified into two types: compound and isolated. Starting now, you should always prioritize compound movements as much as possible when adopting or developing a training plan. However, there should be some room in your program for isolated movements as well. You'll understand why as you learn more about each movement category's specific strengths and weaknesses.

A compound movement is a type of exercise that requires the activation or recruitment of multiple muscle groups located throughout the body. The deadlift is a classic example of such a movement. This necessitates the use of the core muscles, legs, and upper back. The pull-up is another compound movement that requires the use of the biceps, lats, and core. Compound movements are far more beneficial for athletes because they work for multiple muscle groups at once. This means that these movements provide more bang for your buck.

Compound movements also tend to translate better into real-world strength. This means they are more functional in nature and can assist you in improving your performance on daily tasks. A deadlift, for example, can assist you in lifting a large water jug or a piece of furniture off the floor. A pull-up can help you when you need to climb onto an elevated space using only your upper body. Aside from that, compound movements improve your neurological fitness. Because you are working for multiple muscle groups, your brain is also working hard to coordinate the proper function of these different muscle groups.

Isolated movements, as you may have guessed, are exercises that target single muscle groups at a time. They are intended to target only one muscle group, directing all of your attention to that specific area of your body. The bicep curl is a classic example of an isolated movement. A bicep curl, as the name suggests, is a movement that only targets the biceps. The obvious disadvantage of an isolated movement is that you don't get the most bang for your buck. If your training plan consists solely of isolated movements, it will take you much longer to complete a full-body workout. However, this does not rule out the use of isolated movements in your training regimen.

Isolated movements can be extremely effective at achieving specific goals, such as correcting strength imbalances or weaknesses.

This is a topic that will be covered in greater detail later in this chapter.

Holistic Muscle Growth

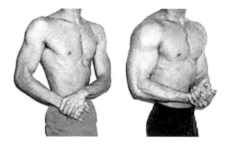

Now it's time to discuss the significance of building your physique holistically. Too often, people avoid working on their weaknesses in favor of focusing solely on their strengths. This isn't limited to the realms of exercise and fitness. It occurs far too frequently in various aspects of life. A writer who is skilled at writing romance will not attempt to write fantasy novels. Boxing-proficient martial artists will be discouraged from participating in wrestling drills. In bodybuilding, a person with strong legs will always prefer squats to pull-ups. As a result, they spend more time doing what they are already good at simply because they enjoy it more. This is the wrong way to build your ideal physique.

One could argue that you should devote more time to your weaknesses to develop your body in a more balanced manner. If you know you are leg-dominant, devote more time and effort to strengthening your upper body. You don't want to end up with elephant legs and toothpick arms, do you? It is critical that you assess your current fitness level before beginning a training program.

Examine yourself in the mirror and conduct an eye test. Do you think your body is proportional? Do your arms appear to be larger than they should be? Is your tummy a little chubby? Do your legs appear to be smaller than the rest of your body? When you determine your strengths and weaknesses, you will have a better idea of what you need to work on when developing your training plan.

Muscle Imbalance Is Dangerous

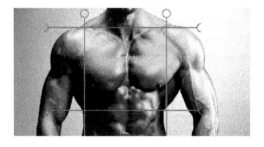

Muscle imbalance is something you must always keep in mind when beginning strength and resistance training.

Too often, whether people are athletes or not, they seek help from therapists or chiropractors for aches and pains in their bodies. These aches and pains are frequently caused by muscle imbalances. Given that you are about to subject your body to a demanding training regimen, you should anticipate that you will be more prone to developing muscle imbalances.

What exactly is Muscle Imbalance?

Simply put, a muscle imbalance occurs when one side of your joint has significantly more strength than the opposing muscle on the opposite side of the joint. This is not how your body should be structured or designed in terms of physiology and biomechanics. When you have a muscle imbalance, this can be considered an abnormality that can lead to serious complications in the way you function biomechanically. When you have strength imbalances throughout your body, one side may end up overcompensating for the other to compensate. This overcompensation may result in injury and tissue damage.

What are the Signs of Muscular Imbalance?

Finding out if you have a muscle imbalance isn't always easy, especially when you're doing it on your own. If you have a trainer watching you while you work out, they may be able to spot weaker areas in your body more easily. However, if you exercise on your own, things may be a little more difficult because you must engage in a high level of self-assessment. Fortunately, there are methods for determining whether you have any existing muscle imbalances. Lower back soreness/pain is one of the most common symptoms of muscle imbalance.

The ache in the neck, impingement of the shoulder, knee discomfort, Rotator cuff tendonitis, joint sprains, tendonitis, slipped discs, muscle tears, and other conditions

Essentially, these kinds of injuries that appear out of nowhere do not exist by chance. They exist for a reason.

You may be wondering what causes these minor aches and pains. They could be the result of a variety of factors. However, you should look into any muscle imbalances you may have.

How Do You Deal with Muscle Imbalances?

Remember how we talked about how compound movements are more efficient at helping you bulk up and get the body you want earlier? That is still the case. However, we also discussed isolated movements and how they contribute to overall strength development. This is where they enter the picture. The most effective way to correct muscle imbalances is to strengthen the weak muscles so that they can catch up with the rest of your body. Isolated movements that target specific muscles are excellent for correcting muscle imbalances.

They are also excellent for providing accessory strength to your more complex compound movements.

For example, while performing a back squat, you may notice that your legs are strong enough to push the weight up, but your core always gives way. You can then perform isolated movements that target specific core muscles to help you improve your back squat. The pull-up is another example of this.

The pull-up is a complex movement that involves many different muscle groups. Some people will struggle to perform a proper pull-up because they are weaker in certain muscle groups. They may have enough let strength to begin the ascent of a pull-up, but not enough bicep strength to complete it. Bicep curls, an isolated movement, can help correct muscle imbalances so that the muscles recruited for pull-up progress are more unified.

Consider your muscles to be a family. Every single muscle group belongs to that family and serves a specific purpose when performing certain movements.

When one member of the family is underperforming, the performance of the entire family suffers. Targeting your muscle imbalances is akin to identifying your family's weakest link and ensuring that they do not fall behind. You should always ensure that all of your muscle groups are progressing at a proportional rate. As unpleasant as it may be,

To confront your weaknesses, you must first address your muscle imbalances before they have any long-term negative effects on your body.

Making a Workout Schedule

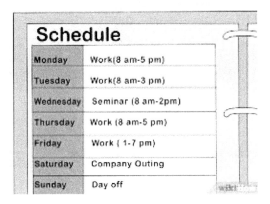

When it comes to structuring your workout plan, remember the various principles we've discussed so far. To refresh, prioritize compound movements to make your workouts and training sessions more efficient.

Next, you should approach muscle building holistically. This means that you should never prioritize one muscle group over another. Finally, you should avoid developing muscle imbalances. This is why you must devise a workout regimen that targets all of your muscle groups and allows them to grow and develop over time.

The first question you may have been how many times per week you should train. The answer, of course, will differ from person to person. Again, it is entirely dependent on your objectives and lifestyle. However, if you're serious about muscle building, you should aim for four to five days of intense training per week.

Again, it takes sheer determination and consistency to achieve the body you desire. If it were simple, everyone would be chiseled. Training sessions should last approximately one hour. If you're quick, you might be able to finish in thirty minutes. It all depends on your level of fitness and how your body reacts to exercise.

Push-Pull Motions

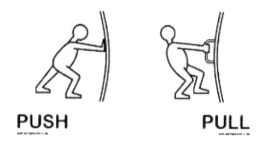

We must also discuss push and pull movements in addition to compound and isolation movements. When it comes to resistance training, your body frequently does one or the other. To lift a weight, you must either push against the force of gravity or pull against the force of gravity. A push-up and a pull-up are two classic examples of this. When selecting the movements that will comprise your workout plan, make sure to include a healthy mix of both push and pull exercises.

You have two options for how you approach this. One option is to dedicate one training session to only push or pull movements and then alternate these sessions throughout the week. Mondays and Wednesdays, for example, could be dedicated to pushing movements, while Tuesdays and Thursdays could be dedicated to pulling movements. Then, on Fridays, you can do a combination of the two. However, incorporating both movements into every training session is another way to structure a push-pull training program. For example, you could schedule six different exercises for Monday. Three of those exercises are push movements, while the other three are pull movements. This exercise format would then be carried throughout the week.

You may be wondering why a push-pull movement or workout plan would benefit you. Finally, the answer can be boiled down to the following reasons:

Provides the Best Recovery
We've already discussed how important rest and recovery are when it comes to muscle building. The push-pull principle of training scheduling can assist you in better structuring your muscle recovery. So, by dividing your training week into different segments (push and pull), you're allowing your muscles to rest on days when they're not active.

For example, if you work on push movements on Monday, you will most likely engage muscle groups such as the quads, pecs, and deltoids. If you focus on pull movements on Tuesday, you are resting Monday's muscles because you are focusing on other muscle groups such as hamstrings, biceps, and lats.

Improves Muscle Balance

By properly dividing a training plan between push and pull movements, the likelihood of developing a muscle imbalance is reduced. When training with the push-pull principle, you must ensure that you are getting equal amounts of each type of movement. If you have three exercises dedicated to push-centric muscles, you should also have three exercises dedicated to pull-centric muscles. This makes it much easier for you to strike that balance when developing your training plans.

Avoids Injuries

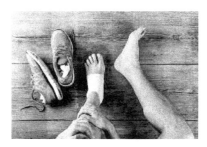

This particular advantage of the push-pull training philosophy is merely a byproduct of the two preceding items.

To begin with, allowing your body ample recovery time in between hard training sessions reduces the likelihood of your body giving up as a result of overtraining. Also, as previously discussed, having a muscle imbalance can make someone more prone to injury.

Because the push-pull style of training reduces the likelihood of developing muscle imbalances, it also eliminates any complications caused by such a condition.

Muscle Building with a Holistic Approach

Push-pull training (when combined with compound movement integration) can help you achieve a more holistic approach to muscle building. You would be able to target multiple muscle groups, ensuring that every area of the body received time and attention.

It saves time.

It makes your workout much more efficient. You don't want to spend all of your time at the gym if you have a day job or a family (unless you're a professional athlete).

Finally, a push-pull philosophy can help simplify the way you structure your training so that you never have to rack your brain trying to figure out what you'll do on any given training day. So, in addition to helping you be more efficient with your time spent at the gym, it also helps you be more efficient when planning your training schedule.

Upper Body Workouts

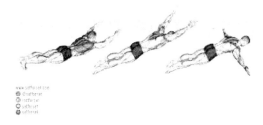

All of the muscles in your arms, upper back, chest, and shoulders are part of your upper body.

Your arms are primarily responsible for lifting yourself onto platforms or moving heavy weight from point A to point B. You can use a variety of upper body exercises in your training plan that is designed to target different muscle groups. Some of the most important compound exercises to incorporate into your routine will be listed here.

Pull-Ups/Chin-Ups (Pull) (Pull)

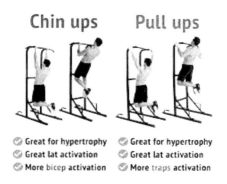

Chin ups | Pull ups

- Great for hypertrophy
- Great lat activation
- More bicep activation

- Great for hypertrophy
- Great lat activation
- More traps activation

Pull-ups are an excellent pulling movement for developing upper body strength. It's a movement that primarily works your biceps. However, depending on how you hold it, it can also help strengthen your biceps and forearms. When you grip the bar with your palms facing you, your biceps are recruited more than your lats.

Variations: Lateral Pull Downs, Supinated Ring Rows

Push-Ups (Push) (Push)

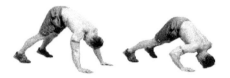

To perform a proper push-up, three major muscle groups must be recruited. One example is the pectoral or chest muscles. The triceps are the muscles located at the back of your upper arm. Finally, there is the front of the shoulders, also known as the deltoids. Push-ups strengthen secondary muscle groups such as the abdomen and the serratus anterior or wings. You can change which muscles are used depending on how your hands are positioned, just like with pull-ups. A wider grip would emphasize the chest, whereas a closer grip would emphasize the triceps.

Push-Ups on a Ledge, Elevated Push-Ups, Handstand Push-Ups, Knee Push-Ups, Dips

Bench Pressing (Push)

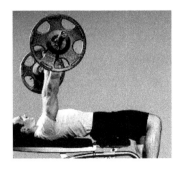

The bench press works similarly to the push-up and recruits the same primary muscle groups. However, because you are not propping your body up, it places less emphasis on the core. A closer grip, like the push-up, recruits the triceps, while a wider grip recruits the chest. This exercise can be done with either dumbbells or barbells.

Bench Press Variations: Inclined Bench Press (Military Press/Shoulder Push)

A military press, also known as a shoulder press, is a movement that can be performed with barbells, dumbbells, or even kettlebells. It primarily targets the deltoids and shoulders, with a secondary emphasis on the triceps. By extension, the movement will recruit the core and legs for added stability, especially if performed standing.

Rows (Pull) (Pull)

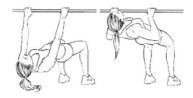

A row is a common exercise that is done with dumbbells or kettlebells. There are, however, variations that allow for the use of barbells. When performing a row, the latissimus dorsi, trapezius, and rhomboid muscles are primarily recruited. Depending on how the grip is positioned, there is also a secondary emphasis on the biceps and forearms.

Variations include bent-over barbell rows and plank rows.

Thrusters are a unique exercise (Push)

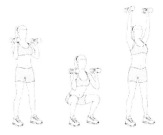

The final upper-body exercise on this list is unique in that it is a full-body movement. Thrusters can be done with a dumbbell, kettlebell, or barbell. It entails combining a weighted squat and a military press in a single swift movement.

Exercises for the Core

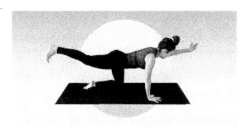

Sure, having a six-pack would feel and look great. But that isn't the most important aspect of having a strong core. Many people do not understand what muscles are involved in core training when they hear the term. They may think of the upper and lower abs, as well as the side obliques, most of the time. Your glutes and lower back are also core muscles in your body. These muscle groups are all responsible for protecting and stabilizing your spine. Without a strong core, your spine is very vulnerable, which can lead to serious injuries, especially when lifting heavy weights. You should always strive to incorporate these fundamental core exercises into your training routine.

Planks

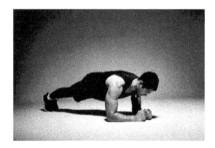

Planks, according to many athletes and coaches, are the most effective way to train your core. This is because the movement effectively recruits every muscle group in your core region. It focuses heavily on your frontal abdomen and lowers your back. A secondary emphasis is placed on your gluteus maximus. There are also plank variations that focus more on the side obliques. As a result, depending on how you hold the plank, the movement can also improve shoulder stability. Side Planks are a variation.

L-Sits

The l-sit is one of the most difficult core exercises to perform because it requires a significant amount of mobility and upper body strength. Most people with tight hips and hamstrings would be unable to perform an l-sit properly due to mobility issues. This is a movement that relies heavily on shoulder stability and pectoral strength for stability. However, raising one's legs to a straight elevated position requires significant abdominal and lower back strength, as well as hip mobility. Hanging L-Sits and Seated L-Sits are two variations.

Raise Your Knees While Hanging

The hanging knee raise is an excellent core exercise that focuses on the frontal abdomen. It is, however, an excellent exercise for increasing grip strength and improving shoulder mobility. The overall goal is to lift the legs by hip-hinging and engaging the core.

Variations: Toes to Bar, Hanging Leg Raise

Back Extenders

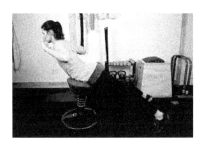

Most core exercises focus primarily on the frontal abdomen, side obliques, or glutes. This is why back extensions are important to include in one's exercise routine because they target the lower back, which is a part of the core muscle groups.

Sit-Ups

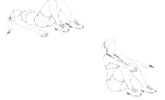

When you think of strengthening someone's abs, your mind goes to Someone performing a series of sit-ups may come to mind. The primary muscle groups that are used for this workout are;

The rectus abdominis, transverse abdominis, and obliques are the muscles involved in a proper sit-up. Sit-ups also help to strengthen the lower back and hip flexors.

Crunches, Butterfly Sit-Ups, and Weighted Sit-Ups are some variations.

Lower Body Workouts

People enjoy flaunting their biceps, back muscles, or abs after a hard workout at the gym. Although you may not realize it, the lower body contains some of the largest muscles in your body. Think about how much you use your legs daily. Whenever you jump, walk, stand, run, or do anything that involves you moving around from one place to the next, you are using your lower body. You wouldn't be as mobile as you are now without your lower extremities. This is why it's important that you pay more attention to training your slower body as well. It isn't just about having the biggest biceps in town. As they say colloquially, don't skip leg day.

Squats (Push) (Push)

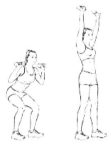

The squat is said to be one of the most important foundational movements that you could ever integrate into your workout routine. Having a strong squat translates to you having stronger legs that will serve as the foundation for whenever you stand, walk, jump, or run. The squat primarily recruits the quadriceps (front area of your leg), but it also has a secondary effect on your glutes, hamstrings, and calves as well.

Variations: Air Squat, Barbell Squat, Pistol Squat, Split Squat

Lunges (Push) (Push)

Lunges are like squats in terms of the muscle groups that they target. However, they offer a greater emphasis on single-leg engagement. This is an effective lower body exercise for addressing strength imbalances between both legs.

Variations: Walking Lunges, Reverse Lunges, Side Lunges

Deadlifts (Pull) (Pull)

If the squat is considered to be one of the most important foundational movements in fitness, then so is the deadlift.

Consider this as a pull variation of the squat, which is a push movement. The deadlift heavily targets the hamstrings, lower back, and glutes. However, it also requires substantial strength around the rest of the core muscles and the legs. Depending on how you position your feet, a deadlift can place heavier emphasis on a specific muscle group.

Variations: Stiff-legged Deadlift, Single-Leg Deadlift, Sumo Deadlift

Calf Raises (Push) (Push)

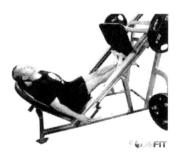

As its name implies, a calf raise is primarily focused on building up the calves. This is a very important exercise for those who are looking to build explosive strength that can translate into better running or jumping. Most leg exercises target the upper leg muscles like the quads and hamstrings. This is why it's important to integrate calf-dedicated exercises like the calf raise into one's bodybuilding routine.

Special Exercise: Cleans (Pull) (Pull)

A clean is also technically a full-body exercise as it is a complex compound movement that recruits various muscle groups. The first phase of a clean is a deadlift that transitions into a powerful hip thrust paired with a violent shrug and pulls from the arms into a strong front rack position. The first phase of as clean recruits the use of all the same muscle groups as a deadlift while the second phase of clean recruits the same muscle groups as that of a row.

The final phase of the catch position of a clean relies on pure core strength to stabilize the barbell.

Variations: Squat Clean, Power Clean, Muscle Clean, Dumbbell Clean

Special Note

Please remember that there are loads of different exercises and movements out there that can't be listed in this book for practicality. Consider the movements listed here to be a list of capsule movements that you should shave to serve as the foundation of your bodybuilding program.

These are the foundational movements that will help you build that starting strength that you need to form good habits at the gym. Over time, as you become more experienced in this field, you will be exposed to more complex variations and modalities. Always feel free to explore these new areas of fitness. Be bold enough to introduce new improvements and rep schemes into your training regimen. This is all a part of the process of testing your body's abilities and seeing just how much you're capable of.

Incorporating Cardio

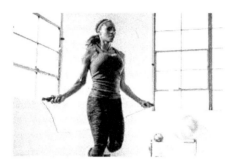

If you're an ectomorph, then try to limit cardio as much as possible. Don't spend more than thirty minutes a week doing cardio. That wouldn't be beneficial to your current fitness goals just yet. If you want to improve your cardiovascular health, then just opt for shorter rest times in between sets while lifting.

This will cause you to have a more elevated heart rate while training and this can also serve as a good exercise for your heart while doing resistance workouts.

If you're a mesomorph, you will need to do more cardio than, an ectomorph, but not so much. Spend around thirty minutes to an hour every week that's dedicated to pure cardio work. Whether it be a jog on the treadmill or a spin class. It's important that you keep your heart healthy and that you do some activities that will help burn away the fat. You have a thriving metabolism and you don't have to worry so much about getting fat unless it's likely that you might be in a constant caloric surplus. Cardio can help make sure that you don't go overboard with your calories so that you don't get any unwanted fat.

If you're an endomorph, as expected, you're going to shave to do the most cardio out of all the body types. Since you're most likely to gain the most pounds, you might have to do a little more work at the gym to burn off some extra calories. You can do 30 minutes of cardio around three to four times a week just to be on the safe side. Again, it doesn't always have to be running on the road or on a treadmill. You can do spin classes, rowers, ellipticals, and other cardio machines. You can also opt to play cardio-heavy sports like basketball, tennis, or football.

Using Supersets

A superset is a common tactic that many lifters will use to introduce an added layer of difficulty and complexity to a workout. Aside from putting more stress on the body as a whole to produce better strength gains, it's also a more efficient way to go about a workout as it minimizes the amount of rest in between exercises. This way, athletes won't have to spend as much time as they need to at the gym.

The way that supersets work is that an athlete performs one set of a particular exercise and then quickly moves on to another set without any time for rest or recovery in between. The idea here is that it keeps the body constantly engaged and it strains the muscles to perform under stress. On top of that, it helps elevate the heart rate while performing resistance training or sexercises that usually don't have a cardiovascular component.

You can make use of the pull-push principle of training into your supersets by putting a push and pull movement against one another. For example, you might be using a squat as the first exercise in the superset. The squat is a push exercise. The next movement would be a row, which is a pull exercise. This is a great way to structure a superset because they offer different stimuli and both exercises recruit different muscle groups. So, while your lower body is recovering from the squats in the first set, you are still putting your body to work by using your upper body to perform the pull-ups.

Sample 1-Week Bodybuilding Program
Based on everything that you've been taught in this chapter so far, it's time for you to create or adopt a training scheme of your own. There are countless resources online that you can tap for ready-made training schemes. But it's also okay if you choose to make one on your own based on the knowledge that you have learned. It's also possible for you to find a ready- \made program and tweak it a little bit so that it accommodates your fitness level.

Here is a sample bodybuilding program that would be good for a week's worth of training. In this sample program, specific days are dedicated to push and pull movements with some days incorporating core training as well. You will also notice that during this exclusive push or pull days, there is a healthy balance between upper body and lower body exercises.

You want to make sure that you are taking a holistic approach to develop your fitness. It's important that you tackle different muscle groups. Also incorporated into this sample program is predetermined and mandatory recovery days. They are mandatory because that means that you have to rest on those days even though you might feel like you can go to the gym and lift. If you're feeling restless, then do some cross-straining.

Again, you shouldn't be training every single day. You need to give ample time for your body to recover in between long stretches of strength training. Feel free to take this sample program and adapt it to your personal preferences.

Monday (Push + Core)
Push-Ups - 3 sets of 12 reps
Barbell Squats - 5 sets of 5 reps
Military Press - 4 sets of 10 reps
Calf Raises - 3 sets of 12 reps
Planks - 3 sets of 1-minute holds
Hanging Leg Raise - 3 sets of 15 reps

Tuesday (Pull) (Pull)
Chin-Ups - 5 sets of 7 reps
Deadlifts - 5 sets of 5 reps
Barbell Rows - 3 sets of 15 reps
Cleans - 5 sets of 3 reps

Wednesday (Push) (Push)
Bench Press - 5 sets of 5 reps
Split Squats - 3 sets of 12 reps (each leg) (each leg)
Dips - 3 sets of 10 reps

Lunges - 3 sets of 12 reps (each leg) (each leg)

Thrusters - 3 sets of 15 reps

Thursday (Active Recovery) Yoga, Swim, Run, Bike, or Mobility Drills

Friday (Pull + Core)

Pull-Ups (or Lateral Pull Down) (or Lateral Pull Down) - 5 sets of 5 reps

Dumbbell Rows - 3 sets of 12 reps

Deadlifts - 5 sets of 5 reps

Toes to Bar - 3 sets of 10 reps

Planks - 3 sets of 1-minute holds

Sit-Ups - 3 sets of 15 reps

Saturday (Active Recovery) Yoga, Swim, Run, Bike, or Mobility Drills

Sunday (Rest) (Rest)

Chapter Six

Progressive Overload

Let's say that you're done with finding a training program that works for you. You've done all of your research and analysis.

You have already scoured the internet for many different workout programs and maybe you've consulted with licensed trainers or coaches to help you make a personalized program.

That's great but the jobs are not done. Learning and research do not stop. Just because you think you have a program that you're ready to start doesn't mean that you're going to be sticking to that program for the rest of your life. As you get better, fitter, and stronger, your workouts are going to feel a lot easier. When that happens, you know that it's time for a change.

One thing you have to know about the journey towards getting fit is that there is no destination. As cliche as it sounds, the journey is the destination. What this means is that the work is never really done. It doesn't matter how fit you become, there is always some work left to do. There is always going to be room for improvement. This is why you should be seeking progress, not perfection.

This chapter is going to help walk you through everything that you need to do AFTER you get started. Of course, getting started is a big step and you should always be proud of that. But it's not just about how you start. Results won't come just because you decide to get better with your fitness. Real results will only come if you continue to stick to the process and stay committed for the long haul.

What is Progressive Overload?

The whole principle of progressive overload centers \around making your workouts more challenging over time. As \you stay consistent with your training and workout regimen, your body is going to go through some amazing changes and transformations. You will find that things that you once found difficult are going to feel a lot easier and simpler to accomplish.

However, while this might seem like good news, it's also going to be detrimental to your progress. The whole point of working out is challenging your muscles to the point of breakage so that there is ample space for growth and development. When there are fewer challenges, then there is also less room for growth.

Think of a first-grade student who is just being introduced to basic math. They learn about addition and subtraction. They might even learn about multiplication and division. As they learn about these concepts, they are making substantial strides from when they first started. Over time, with enough practice, they get better at developing their mathematical skills to the point where these concepts no longer prove to be challenging. When that sharpens, their growth stops. This is why second-grade students will then be introduced to the world of fractions and percentages.

This is to add another layer of complexity and challenge to the students and by extension, it also expands their room for growth.

It's the same as when you work out. Progressive overload isn't a principle that is only applicable to strength training or resistance training. If you're a runner, you practice progressive overload by increasing the speed or distance of your runs. This is a concept that can be applied to so many different disciplines. It's all because it promotes perpetual growth and development by continually introducing newer and more challenging stimuli.

How Does it Benefit Your Training?

One thing that you should expect to experience whenever you engage in resistance training is a plateau. The success that you get from working out is going to deliver some very remarkable results. However, this success that you gain isn't always going to be linear in its rate of growth. There is a good chance that the fitter you get, then the smaller your gains will end up being. Ultimately, it might even get to a point where your body will begin to plateau. This means that you are no longer getting any gains or experiencing any progress whatsoever.

The main reason for this plateau can often be attributed to your rate of effort. The fitter you get, then the less effort is required of you to complete certain physical tasks.

Pushing a 135-pound barbell overhead is going to be a lot more difficult at the start compared to when you're six or eight weeks into your training program. This is because you're getting fitter and the workouts are becoming easier. When your workouts get easier, you aren't pushing your muscles to the point of breakage anymore. This is why progressive overload is the biggest tool that you can use to help combat whatever plateaus you might encounter on your road to fitness.

How Does Progressive Overload Work?
The concept of progressive overload is relatively simple.

It's just a matter of you trying to find ways to make your workouts more challenging as you get fitter. Again, the fitter you get, the better you become at working out. This means that certain workouts that you did two or three weeks ago may no longer be as challenging now as when you first did them. So, you need to change these workouts up a bit to make sure that the stimulus still provides your body with a proper challenge. Now, how do you go about doing so? Well, there are three different approaches that you could take to introducing progressive overload into your training routine.

Increase Resistance
The first way to progressively overload yourself is to increase the level of resistance of your strength training. For example, let's say week one of the programs had you deadlifting a barbell for five sets of five reps at 225 lbs. You repeat this cycle for maybe another week or two. Then, in the third or fourth week, you might find that these sets are a lot easier to accomplish, and you're no longer challenged by them. You can make the exercise smore challenging by increasing resistance or adding weight. In this case, you can up the weight to 235 lbs. This progressive overload is

meant to adapt to your changing and improving level of fitness. Now, you might wonder about how much weight you should be adding. Well, it's going to be different for everyone as people tend to progress differently as well. However, a good rule of thumb to follow is that you should never look to increase the weight beyond 10% of what you were capable of lifting a week prior.

Increase Volume (Reps)

If you don't want to increase resistance, another way that you can go about introducing progressive overload is by increasing the volume of your workouts. If we stick to the same example of deadlifts at 225 lbs., you can still choose to keep the exercise at that weight as you get fitter. However, to progressively overload your system, you might want to increase the volume. So, try adding another set or a few extra reps for every set into your routine. Instead of five sets of five reps, maybe you can do six sets with the same rep scheme. You could also choose to stick to the same five sets, but with seven reps for each set now.

Increase the Rate of Work

Lastly, you could also opt to just increase your rate of work or productivity when you lift. Again, let's just stick to the same example of deadlifts at 225 lbs. for consistency. In the first week, it might have taken you around a full two or three minutes to recover in between each set. If you want to progressively overload yourself by increasing your rate of work, you can minimize the amount of rest that you take in between sets. By the fourth week, maybe your rest period in between sets would be around one minute to 90 seconds long instead of the two to three minutes you took when you first started.

Even making this simple tweak can introduce a new stimulus to your body's muscular system and will offer the benefits of progressive overloads.

Rules of Progressive Overload

By now, you should already have a good idea of what progressive overload is, why it's important, and how you're supposed to execute it. It's always good if you want to continue to introduce your body to new challenges, but you always have to be careful in doing so. By exposing your body to increasingly stressful environments, you have to make sure that you are keeping yourself safe and protected at all times. Progressive overload doesn't mean you going big whenever you're feeling confident. You still have to be methodical and tactical about it. Here are a few rules that you need to keep in mind when practicing progressive overload.

Always Start with Perfect Form

First of all, progressive overload should not even be an option for you if you're lifting with imperfect form. Again, if your form is bad, it doesn't matter how much weight you're lifting. You're doing sit wrong and you're not going to get the gains that you want. Lifting with proper form means that you're engaging the proper muscle groups and that you're hitting all the right spots when it comes to your body's range of motion. If you can't perfect your form at lower weights or rep schemes, it wouldn't be wise for you to be progressing towards more challenging variations. There's no need to rush the process of progressive overload after all. Only move on when you're truly ready to do so.

Progressive Overload is Not a Linear Process

When you first start working out, you might think that you need to put pressure on yourself to just keep on improving and improving at a rapid rate. You might create a schedule for yourself about how much you should be lifting at a certain date.

This is the wrong approach. You have to understand that your gains can't be scheduled. You shouldn't be giving yourself deadlines on how much weight you can lift. Progressive overload is something that you can only execute depending on what your body is capable of handling. It's not some kind of schedule that you NEED to adhere to for it to be effective. If your body is not capable of moving \son from a particular level of resistance or volume, then stay at that level for a while.

Strength Gains Decrease Over Time and Increased Ability

Lastly, you have to expect that progressive overload is not going to become as rampant the older and more experienced you become in this field of fitness. When you're just starting, you will likely experience significant jumps in your strength and abilities. This means that your progressive overload cycles might be a little more frequent. You might be lifting significantly more weight in just a matter of one week.

However, the more experienced and fitter you become, these strength gains become less and less frequent. Some serious lifters out here might even have to train a full year just to be able to gain s5 extra pounds on a single lift.

Chapter Seven

Final Tips to Remember

We're nearly reaching the end of the road here. You've come so far, but you still have far left to go. Fortunately, you know that you don't have to do everything on your own. Granted, this book might have been overwhelming to consume if you read it all at once. However, you will find that over time, with consistent practice, the knowledge in this book will become second nature to you. You might be able to write your book on this topic one day. For now, just try to absorb little bits and pieces as much as you can and integrate these tidbits of knowledge into your daily training.

To conclude this book, here are a few key tips that you might want to keep to heart as you make your way through your fitness journey. Consider these tips to be the summary of everything that you've learned so far.

Don't Overtrain

Always make sure that you never overtrain. This means that you need to devote some time out of your training week to rest and recovery. Sure, you might think that doing more work will lead to more gains. That principle works only to a certain extent.

Doing excessive work will not lead to gains. Rather, it will only lead to unwanted injuries that will sideline you and leave you worse off than when you started. Yes, you want to be giving it your best, but you don't want to overstretch yourself. In this case, it's better to work smarter than it is to work harder.

Leave Your Ego at the Door

One big mistake that amateur lifters or athletes make when they first start is that they let their pride get to them.

Sometimes, their pride will lead to them thinking that they're capable of lifting more weight than they can. What ends up happening? Injuries. Sometimes, their pride will have them believe that they are better or fitter than other people in the gym.

This is the completely wrong mindset to have when approaching fitness. Your only goal at the gym every time you go there is to be better than the person that you were yesterday. Focus on that and the results will come.

Stay Consistent

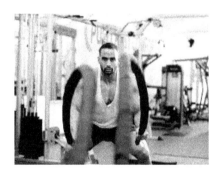

Remember that old story about the tortoise and the hare?

It's cool to be fast, but slow and steady wins the race. If you think that you can just go to the gym once or twice a week and give your maximum effort for every session to get your desired results, then you would be mistaken. It would be a lot better for you to go to the gym multiple times a week and give small, but consistent efforts during every session. Eventually, these small efforts will add up to substantial gains that will only be given to you in the long run.

Don't Under eat

Even if you're an endomorph who is prone to gaining weight, it's important that you don't undereat. Of course, it should be obvious as to why an ectomorph shouldn't be undereating.

Food is your friend, not your enemy. You need food to generate the fuel that is necessary for you to work hard at the gym. Without food, your muscles will not be able to grow and perform as efficiently as they should. It's all about moderation.

You don't want to overeat, that's true, but it's just as important that you don't undereat.

Keep Hydrated

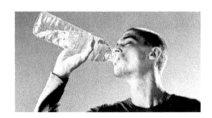

Stay hydrated at all times. Whether you're a serious athlete or not, you need water to survive. When you put in all of that effort in your training, you're going to break a lot of sweat. You should never feel dehydrated as a result of your workout. Water also helps your body function properly, particularly when it comes to processing nutrients from food. Water will aid in the protein synthesis process, which is intended to aid in muscle growth.

Prioritize Getting Enough Sleep

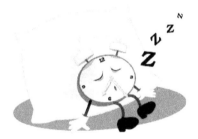

Sleep is an underappreciated resource that many people take for granted. As a bodybuilder, you subject your body to a great deal of stress. This is why you, more than most other people, require more sleep. When you sleep at night, your body is working double-time to revitalize and repair itself. Also, sleep allows you to regain energy, which will fuel you for another day of hard training.

Lift with proper form at all times.

This is something that far too many gym rats do. Even people who have been working out for years can make this critical error. Some people will compromise their form to complete a workout faster or lift heavier weights. This is a huge mistake because bad lifting form (especially when the weights get heavy) can result in serious life-threatening injuries. You should never attempt a PR back squat without first bracing your core. This is the quickest way to injure your spine and potentially paralyze yourself.

Exercise is not inherently dangerous, and you should not be afraid of it. You simply must ensure that you are lifting with proper form every time to keep yourself safe and protected.

Do Only the Appropriate Amount of Cardio

Cardio is a subject that has been covered extensively in this book. Again, there is no set volume or amount of cardio that everyone should do every day or week. It all depends on your physiological makeup and personal objectives.

However, as a general rule, if you want to build muscle, you should focus on resistance training while limiting aerobic activities like running. This is especially true if you are an ectomorph who has difficulty gaining weight. A significant amount of cardio may be counterproductive to your goals.

Stop Comparing Your Success to the Success of Others.

The most important thing to remember about your fitness journey is that it is entirely your responsibility. Unless you're discussing your trainer, coach, or therapist, your health and wellness goals are not the concern of others. The same can be said for you. Don't make fun of someone at the gym who isn't progressing as quickly as you are. They are on their fitness journey, and it is unimportant to you. It's the same when you see someone you believe is doing better than you. Just because they appear to be more successful does not mean that your success is invalid. Be content with your accomplishments and move on. Stop measuring yourself against others.

Supplements Should Not Be Feared

Finally, don't be afraid to use supplements. Whey protein, on the other hand, is not a steroid. Creatine is not a performance-enhancing substance. Supplements contain essential nutrients similar to those found in the food you eat every day. Supplements, on the other hand, should be viewed as supplemental products to your diet. Finally, your diet should consist of whole foods such as meats, vegetables, fruits, and grains. You should only use supplements when you feel you need a few extra nutrients that you can't get from natural food.

Conclusion

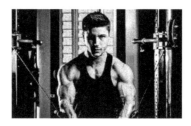

We've arrived at the end. Hopefully, this book has motivated you to begin strength training. At the very least, it should have increased your motivation to become the best version of yourself possible. Yes. You deserve to have the body you desire. Fitness is not a privilege or a luxury reserved only for those who will benefit from it.

Fitness is a right that you must earn through willpower, dedication, and hard work. It may not always be easy to achieve fitness, but it is always possible. It makes no difference what your background is. Whether you grew up in an athletic family or not, you are capable and deserving of pursuing and achieving your own fitness goals.

Too many people around the world make the mistake of believing that they cannot succeed. That is rarely the case. Improving one's fitness is a goal that can be attained by almost anyone. Even people with physical disabilities can strive to be better versions of themselves.

People do not lack opportunities to become more fit. What they lack is the commitment and willpower to pursue these objectives.

You may have been guilty in the past of making numerous excuses for not making time for fitness. You were too preoccupied. You were under the impression that you didn't have enough time. You didn't have enough money to join a gym. These are all kinds of excuses that people have been using for a long time. Finally, you should realize that you will never hear excuses from people who genuinely want to make changes in their lives. This is because those who are truly committed to making these changes will not be preoccupied with making excuses. Rather, they concentrate on solutions. You are demonstrating to yourself that you are shifting your focus toward the solution by reading this book. You recognize that there is a problem and that your life could be better. The fact that you're looking for solutions indicates that you're ready to take the next big step.

Remember that on your journey to fitness, you will inevitably make mistakes. Success will not come to you immediately, and when it does, it will not always be linear. You will have your share of ups and downs, just like in life. Now and then, you might feel like you're taking two steps forward and one step back. That's fine. That is completely normal. Slumps and setbacks of this magnitude are to be expected. They aren't nearly as important as how you react to such occurrences whenever they occur.

Remember that one of the most important qualities you must cultivate here is persistence. There will always be numerous reasons why you should not exercise. There will be numerous factors out there that will discourage you from pursuing your dreams. You will undoubtedly encounter a few roadblocks that will make you want to give up. But if you stick with it long enough, none of this will matter. They will only be a minor stumbling block on your path to self-actualization.

As you go out and put forth the effort to get the body of your dreams, always remember that you are worthy of having such dreams in the first place. Be proud of yourself for believing that you deserve to be a better version of yourself. This is advantageous not only to you but also to those who will view your work. You will be a beacon of hope and inspiration to those who are afraid to begin. Those who don't believe in themselves will find empowerment and confidence in your spirit. That is also one of the best aspects of fitness. It's a neighborhood. Even if you have your own goals and mostly work out alone, you are aware that there are others out there who are going through the same things you are. Others have equally lofty ambitions and goals. Having that knowledge alone will provide you with a sense of solidarity from others in the fitness community to continue pursuing your goals. And by actively participating in the community, you are effectively doing the same for those around you.

I'm Baz Thompson, the founder of CJD Fitness and a CYQ Master Personal Trainer who has helped hundreds of people just like you achieve their fitness goals. I coach global executives and people of all ages, as well as professional athletes. and I have appreciated the opportunity to work with you.

Finally, if you have benefited from reading this book and believe that others who have reached or passed the age of 40 and want to get in shape could benefit as well, please consider leaving a positive review on Amazon. This will send a message to other potential readers in need of assistance and reassure them that this book is for them.

I hope you have excellent health and well-being on your long journey through life, and I wish you all the best. Thank you for allowing me to share my expertise with you.

.

CPSIA information can be obtained
at www.ICGtesting.com
Printed in the USA
BVHW051402270223
659294BV00014B/570